DON'T BE FOOLED

DON'T BE FOOLED

Be Conscious Fountain of Youth

GAUTAM KAPUR

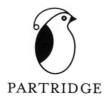

PARTRIDGE

Print information available on the last page.

To order additional copies of this book, contact
Partridge India
000 800 10062 62
orders.india@partridgepublishing.com

www.partridgepublishing.com/india

BE CONSCIOUS IS IN THE BUSINESS OF HEALTHY FOODS AVAILABLE THROUGH TOP ONLINE MARKETPLACES LIKE www.amazon.in/www.ebay.in/www.beconscious.in & others

THE FOOD YOU EAT CAN BE EITHER......
THE SAFEST & MOST POWERFUL FORM
OF NATURAL MEDICINE
OR
THE SLOWEST FORM OF POISON
- ANN WIGMORE

Contents

Chapter 1. Introduction 1

Chapter 2. Go Get That Knowledge And Turbo Charge Your Life 7

Chapter 3. Overweight and Obesity 17

Chapter 4. Mind and Body Connection 32

Chapter 5. Sleep 36

Chapter 6. Super Foods 46

Chapter 7. A Few Food Demons 72

Chapter 8. A Simple Formula for Healthy Living:
70% Kitchen, 30% Exercise 74

Chapter 9. Are Your Hormones Causing You Havoc? 83

Chapter 10. Definition of Concepts 86

BE CONSCIOUS (Recommended) DIET 101

Chapter One

Introduction

One cannot think well, love well, and sleep well, if one has not dined well
- Virginia Woolf

It is an established fact even from elementary school that the effect of food on the body cannot be quantified as we all need food to survive. As a matter of fact, even parents emphasize it when they try to get the children to eat healthy. So it would probably be safe to say it is a cliché how much our nutritional lifestyle affects our health. An article published by the University of Minnesota likened the food we eat to giving our body information and materials they need to function properly. If we don't get the right information, our metabolic processes suffer and our health declines. And for some rather perplexing reason, the world in reference to nutrition seems to forget or maybe just ignore the mortality of man. Many people prefer to live in the moment and so whatever they crave at any particular moment is gobbled up without qualms. The problem with this is not so much being spontaneous, as the right kind of spontaneity. You can be impulsive with the place to travel to, where to have fun but when your health is in question, you cannot afford to be impulsive. There is a lot to be said for having a clear-cut plan about how and what you eat, unless of course you are not so psyched about living the next adventure out.

It is against this background that it becomes expedient to monitor how we eat by checking the nutrients we get from everything we eat. This might sound like too much work, but it is definitely better than spending life savings on a sickness that could have been prevented just by eating right. There is no substitute for eating right in our body's metabolism. Other things are necessary and even important, but only nutrients can do some things for you. A sage once said, "If you do not make food your medicine, you would one day make medicine your food." What this simply means is that just as you are asked to take medication carefully and with the right dosage, so are we expected to eat, using the right dosage, which in this case is a well-balanced diet. Or else, one is likely to get sick; Medication becomes a normal and natural part of that person for the rest of his/her life. The authors of *Perspective in Nutrient* described nutrients as "the nourishing substances in food that are essential for the growth, development and maintenance of body functions." This essentially means that if a nutrient is not present, aspects of function and therefore human health decline. When nutrient intake does not regularly meet the nutrient needs dictated by the cell activity, the metabolic processes slow down or even stop. It is therefore a non- negotiable deal that nutrients are basic in the life of a man and should not be taken with levity or worse, considered unimportant. We should make it a point to change if we haven't earlier thought to do so.

CAN YOU FIND A CORNER IN A ROUND ROOM? – WELL YOU CAN'T, CAN YOU?

Change is probably one of the most difficult things to do, but it is also most times the best thing to do. Change requires development and moving from the past ways of doing things, requires leaving your comfort zone and taking risks. Therefore, it could be very uncomfortable and challenging. But we have already established that sometimes, it is necessary. Thus, it has to be done, most especially in the area of food. Have the/your fundamental choices of food changed? If NOT you are in that very Round room going around in circles. The quote by Aristotle comes to mind here that *"WE ARE WHAT WE REPEATEDLY DO"*, and we can extend it to say we are what we eat. What we eat over an amount of time accumulates and produces result; good or bad.

ONLY CHANGE CAN BRING ABOUT CHANGE

So if we want to see changes, we are going to have to make changes. It is not enough to watch 'the biggest loser on television,' hoping that one day you would get the opportunity to be on the reality show so you can lose some weight. As a matter of fact, some people would most probably be eating that heavyweight burger while watching the show and prepared to be seated throughout the day in front of the television. And they wonder why the people on screen look *FIT AND HEALTHY.* Why not take a cue from 'biggest loser' and even from your home try some of the things they are doing to keep yourself in shape? If you do not make a conscious decision to change, chances are you would keep moving in circles, and you would be the exact person who is looking for a corner in a round room.

Look around you, there is so much junk food. The system allows it and your system fails to resist it and eventually pays the price for it with toxic medication & ridiculous hospital bills. So bring into balance this excessive energy and come back to your axis. BE CONSCIOUS!

Do not be deceived; you cannot find a corner in a round room till you build a room with four corners or edges. What this means is you can continue to look at people giving in to exercises and good nutrition and wish you were in their position; that would not get you there. If wishes were horses, beggars would ride. Unfortunately for us as much as we would have hoped it was, wishes are not horses, it is actually actions that bring about results. Wishes only bring results in fairy tales and the world of make-believe. In real life, everybody you see with changes actually worked hard at it. You can do the same. Only work can bring about change, knowledge when applied is freedom/ liberation, while unapplied knowledge is a burden - you are carrying The Demon on your back. Your knowledge, no matter how vast cannot help you. Wisdom as awesome as it sounds does not mean anything abstract. It actually simply means application of knowledge. You are wise if you apply all the knowledge you have on health, nutrition and lifestyle and not just keep storing them.

IT IS BETTER TO LET BAD FOOD GO TO WASTE THAN TO YOUR WAIST

I know you are a conservationist and it irks you to see things go to waste. You would literally do anything to save food from going to waste. Now, here is the bummer, as much as it pains you to let food go to waste, it is necessary for your health and even the world in totality to let some food go to waste. You would be saving yourself from a whole lot of trouble if you just let it go. Sure most of us want that juicy burger but your stomach is not a dumping ground, and it doesn't have to be you that would end up with that burger. Let it go! Give it up! I know it hurts but deep inside *YOU wants YOU* to be healthy.

It is a lot better for everybody involved that the food goes to waste than for it to end in your waist. What that would mean in such situation in case you do not know is that it increases your weight, increases the level of bad cholesterol and triglycerides in the body, which in turn causes all these chronic diseases that the world is battling with. Diabetes, angina, lupus, heart diseases, cancer, Alzheimer disease and so many more could begin to creep in as a result of not letting food go to waste.

On the other hand, you would not want foods like fruits and green vegetables to go to waste. Those ones are protective and good for you. They save you from chronic illnesses and keep you healthy. It just so happens that 90% of the time, when people do not want to waste food, they are talking about junks and unhealthy foods. We would not have so many problems if the foods in question were healthy. So the point is that we should watch for our weight and make sure we are healthy and allow foods that are risk factors of various fatal diseases go to waste.

INDULGE AND YOU WILL BULGE

Has it ever occurred to you that the way to stay healthy is to stay away from those things that are likely to cause us harm? If we look closely, we would discover that man has always flouted rules that would benefit him as a man. But there is truth in a proverb that says, "forbidden fruit is sweet, but the aftermath is most often bitter." All these junk foods are attractive and they are easy "go to" meals especially when you get back from work and the last thing you feel like doing is taking the time out to prepare a healthy home cooked meal. Just remember that forbidden food is sweet, but the aftermath is often bitter, just remember that you could always indulge yourself but be ready to deal with the bulge that follows. Everything we do has consequences, no matter what it is. So if indulging in sweets and junk has become your norm, be ready to let bulges become your norm as well. You do not sow mangoes and get oranges; you get exactly what you give. So if you want to live healthy, then you have to work towards it and avoid things that would prevent you from getting what you want.

BE KIND TO YOURSELF

It is really your choice whether to effect changes in your world or not. If you are reading this, you are probably an adult and in charge of your choices. So nobody can really force you to do anything you don't want to do. However, this is different from entreating you to do something that is difficult and of little benefit to you. While taking care of your diet might be difficult, but it is of immense benefit to you. And as a matter of fact, there have been new discoveries, and it is now possible to make healthy meals interesting. So you do not have to deal with boring diets just to stay healthy. You could make your food interesting yet healthy. For example, instead of dealing with bland meals, you could stock up your kitchen with healthy options like seeds, nuts, and other munchies when you feel like snacking. Make yourself a few healthy salad & snack options, readily available for you to eat when you are hungry instead of grabbing anything that is within your reach "*BECOME A FOOD NINJA.*"

The point of all the above is that alternative has been provided to make making a lifestyle changes an easy decision. But whatever the case, you have to remember that it is about you and nobody else. It is about making you a better you and keeping you in good shape. Be kind to yourself. Understand your food habits and learn to differentiate between your Foodie *NEEDS & DESIRES*. There is a huge difference between what you want to eat and what you need to eat. In the concept of the scale of preference in economics, needs are usually differentiated from wants. Wants are those things one desires to have, but are not basic or have no relative effect on one's survival. Needs on the other hands are basic and major factors in one's survival. Since the beginning of time, we know that wants and needs have always been in a huge conflict with each other. Whereas it should be natural that we discard our wants for our needs, ironically, what we do instead is concentrate on our wants at the expense of our needs. And you know the shocker? We would suffer the consequences and not somebody else. Likewise with our food, we forget that concentrating so much on our wants and desires is the root cause of the overweight problem and obesity that our world is battling with. According to the National Institute of Diabetes and Digestive and Kidney Diseases, more than two-thirds (68.8 percent) of adults are considered to be overweight or obese, more than one-third (35.7 percent) of adults are considered to be obese, and more than 1 in 20 (6.3 percent) have extreme obesity. This is such an alarming statistic and if care is not taken, it would increase as the years go by. That is the reason why to avoid being part of the statistics; we need to take extra care. We need to be deliberate about making changes. As a point of emphasis, it is about you, be kind to yourself, take care of your body; you only have one of it.

Chapter Two

Go Get That Knowledge And Turbo Charge Your Life

*Eating is not merely a material pleasure. Eating well gives a
spectacular joy to life and contributes immensely to goodwill and
happy companionship. It is of great importance to the morale*
- Elsa Schiaparelli

After all that has been said, you really cannot do much if you have no knowledge of what to do. Much knowledge abounds about how important a lifestyle change is but not as much is available about what to do or even how food really affects us. Most people only know the periphery and have not been fortunate to go beyond the surface of nutrition. Equipping yourself with valuable knowledge with regards to your health is equally as important as the willingness to make changes.

Nutrition according to the dictionary is the process of absorbing nutrients from food and the processing by the body in order to keep healthy or to grow. A balanced diet, on the other hand, is a way of eating all of the right nutrients that your body needs in order to be healthy. Those basic nutrients needed in the body include carbohydrates, proteins, minerals, vitamins, fats and oil, and water in the **right proportion**. Now, it is not really taking in the nutrients that is the problem but identifying the right proportion. Most times we dwell more on a particular nutrient at the expense of the others. And some are needed in more proportions than the others, but it is to be noted that there is none of them that are not necessary for the body.

CARBOHYDRATES

So let me explain, many of us have this belief that Carbohydrates should be avoided if you need to lose weight and for various other reasons. "CARBS" are vital and are needed for energy production. Let's break down this BIG word CARBOHYDRATES PHEW! It's actually quite simple: CARBO = CARBON, HYDRE= HYDROGEN & ATE= OXYGEN. So you see these are important sources of energy. Foods such as rice, spaghetti, yams, bread, potatoes, noodles, snacks made with flour and cereals contain starch and are therefore Carbohydrates.

A STARCHY FACT: Starch is converted to Glucose & glucose zips around in the blood and is used by our tissues for energy production. Another widely used CARB is Sucrose (Sugar) that we use dangerously and is present in way too many beverages and today's foods. *MY ADVICE: TREAD CAREFULLY WITH THIS ONE!*

During digestion or as part of the digestive process, all the starch is converted to another form called glucose. Glucose is carried around the body in the blood and is used by our tissues as a source of energy. Any glucose in our food is absorbed without the need for digestion. We also get some of our carbohydrates in the form of sucrose; this is the sugar which we put in our tea and coffee. This is the reason why sugar is not considered healthy because it comes in the original form and the body doesn't process it, leading a lot of times to excesses. Sugar is the highest root cause of obesity and some other diseases like heart diseases, diabetes and so on in the society because it is practically in everything that is considered as standard diet. Medical practitioners says we should make sure our daily intake of energy comes from carbohydrates but for a sedentary lifestyle, you would need less considering you are not burning the energy.

PROTEINS

Proteins is the source of materials for growth and repair. They are in charge of all the repairs that our body undergoes, for instance, if you have an injury, proteins help you fight and heal the injury, and they also repair worn out tissues in the body. Proteins contain carbon, hydrogen, oxygen, nitrogen and occasionally, Sulphur. Proteins need to be turned into Amino acids for digestion as they consist of large molecules so they cannot get directly into our blood. An interesting point is our bodies can also convert the amino acids back into protein. In the event of excesses, amino acids are removed from the body as nitrogen is flushed out as urea. The production of urea happens in the Liver and the Kidney's role is now to put the urea into our urine. This goes to show that excess protein is not as dangerous as excess carbohydrates. However, that does not mean we can be complacent and bombard our system with protein: if the kidneys are overworked, they could break down and that would result into another chronic disease. Nutritionists recommend a fairly modest protein intake. However, it also still depends on the activity level, gene, body weight and all other factors. Therefore for an average sedentary man, 56 grams per day is recommended and 46 grams per day for an average sedentary woman. Food sources include; eggs, milk, yogurt, fish and seafood, soya, pistachio, nuts, pork, chicken and turkey.

FATS AND OIL

Fats are also an energy source and contain fat soluble vitamins like carbohydrates,

FATS = Carbon, Hydrogen and Oxygen.

FATS help and keep us insulated from the cold. Excess Carbohydrate and Protein intake will cause the body to convert some of it into fat. So if you eat too much carbs and proteins in the first place, you would need to drastically reduce your fats intake or better still, you would need to reduce the others to keep your diet balanced or else, you will put on weight. So the Key is to balance your food intake with your exercise regimen or output. However, keep in mind that some fats in your diet is important because the body requires the fat soluble vitamins. For a sedentary lifestyle, stick to about 84 to 85 grams of fats or less to stay healthy. Food sources include; salmon, nuts and seeds, plant oils, and avocadoes.

VITAMINS

Vitamins are only required in very small quantities. There is no chemical similarity between these chemicals; the similarity between them is entirely biological.

Vitamin A (Retinol): good for your eyes, for example, sweet potatoes, carrots, spinach, fortified cereals, etc.

Vitamin B: They consist of about 12 different chemicals;

- Vitamin B1 (Thiamine): helps the body process some carbohydrates and protein, for example, whole-grain, enriched, fortified products like bread and cereals, etc.
- Vitamin B2 (Riboflavin): helps make red blood cells, for example, milk, bread products, fortified cereals, etc.
- Vitamin B3 (Niacin): helps with digestion and with making cholesterol, for examples, meat, fish, poultry, enriched and whole grain breads, fortified cereals, etc.
- Vitamin B5 (Pantothenic Acid): helps turn carbohydrates, protein, fats into energy, for example, chicken, beef, potatoes, oats, cereals, tomatoes, etc.
- Vitamin B6 (Pyridoxine): helps with metabolism, the immune system and also the development of baby's brain, for example, fortified cereals, fortified soy products, chickpeas, potatoes, organ meats, etc.
- Vitamin B7 (Biotin): helps the body to make fat, protein and any other nutrients the cells need, for example, liver, fruits, meats, etc.
- Vitamin B8 (Inositol): controls hypertension, helps to reduce depression and other psychological disorders, for example, beef, egg yolk, cereals, rice, citrus fruits, green leafy vegetables, molasses, soy nuts, etc.

- Vitamin B9 (Folic Acid): it helps prevent birth defect, helps digestion, build healthy red blood cells, for example, leafy green vegetables and enriched grains.
- Vitamin B12 (Cobalamin): helps the body make red blood cells, for example, fish, poultry, meat, dairy products, fortified cereals, etc.
- Vitamin C (Ascorbic Acid): needed for your body to repair itself, for example, red and green peppers, kiwis, oranges and other citrus fruits, strawberries, broccoli, tomatoes, etc.
- Vitamin D (The Sunshine Vitamin): can be made in your skin, needed for absorption of Calcium, for example, fish liver oils, fatty fish, fortified milk products, fortified cereals, etc.
- Vitamin E (Tocopherols and Tocotrienols): is implicated in many of the body's processes, for example, fortified cereals, sunflower seeds, almonds, peanut butter, vegetable oils, etc.
- Vitamin K: important in blood clotting and bones maintenance, for example, Green vegetables like spinach, collards, and broccoli; Brussels sprouts; cabbage, etc.

MINERALS

Minerals are also needed in small quantities, but we need more of these than we need of vitamins. The body is a vast chemical reaction system with millions of different reactions all going on producing the substances that we need to survive. If we are lacking any of the vitamins and minerals, then these reactions cannot continue and we become ill. They include;

Iron: required to make hemoglobin, for examples, fortified cereals, beans, lentils, beef, turkey (dark meat), soy beans, spinach, etc. Calcium: required for healthy teeth, bones and muscles, for example, soy milk, yogurt, hard cheeses, fortified cereals, kale, etc.

Choline: needed to make cells, for example, milk, liver, eggs, peanuts, etc.

Folic Acid: helps prevent birth defects, important for heart health and for cell development, for example, dark, leafy vegetables; enriched and whole grain.

Iodine: used to make a hormone called thyroxin, for example, seaweed, seafood, dairy products, processed foods, iodized salt, etc.

Sodium: all cells need this, especially nerve cells, important for food balance. It is found in foods made with added salt.

There are several other trace elements that are essential such as copper, magnesium, phosphorus and selenium. These are often implicated in enzyme catalysis for very important reactions.

WATER

Water has been proven to be very necessary and we should take a lot. It is commonly recommended to drink eight 8-ounce glasses of water per day. After all, water makes up about two thirds of who we are, and influences 100 percent of the processes in our body. About 60 percent of the body is made of water. Drinking enough water maintains the body's fluid balance, which helps transport nutrients in the body, regulate body temperature, helps control calories, helps energizes the muscles, cleanses the kidney, maintains bowel function among other functions.

From the above, we can see clearly that we need to have all the nutrients in our diet to live healthy but the trick is having it in the right proportion. Nothing is good about excesses, so it should be largely discouraged. And deficiency would also not do us any good. A lot of people because of how much they have heard about the amount of calories in carbohydrates would decide to stay away from carbohydrates so they can lose weight and some because they are diabetic. The best that could happen if you want to lose weight is that you do lose some weight but you become lethargic and in a worst situation, there is a breakdown of the body system. And in the case of the diabetic patient, you could have low blood sugar, which at its peak is even more lethal than high blood sugar at its peak. The key is balance.

Learning or knowing about the basics of nutrition boils down to understanding the roles that specific nutrients play in a healthy diet. Globally, there is an increased mortality rate compared to a century ago and even decades ago. Life expectancy has drastically reduced, especially in the third world countries (this fact on life expectancy and mortality rate is an average estimation). And for most nations in the world, a bulk of the portion of the budget apportioned to health goes to chronic diseases. Initially, medical practitioners explained all these chronic diseases on the genes. There was a wide spread belief that for one to be prone to a particular disease depends largely on the genes, on whether the family he is from has a history of that disease. While this theory has not been discarded, it has been discovered through rigorous research that the food we eat has more to do with these diseases. Specific dietary factors have been associated with the cause or prevention of conditions as diverse as cancer, coronary heart disease, birth defects, and Cataracts. To prevent the onset of these diseases, we need to know how multiple nutrients in a diet interact and affect the human body's functions, according to the *Nutrition Society*, Europe's largest nutritional organization. Therefore, in C. Willett's article, *'Diet and Health: What Should We Eat?'* the recommendations of NRC based on their discovery of the relation between health and diet. They recommended that;

1. Reduce total fat intake to 30% or less of calories. Reduce saturated fatty acid intake to less than 10% of calories and the intake of cholesterol to less than 300 mg daily.

2. Every day, eat five or more servings of a combination of vegetables and fruits, especially green and yellow vegetables and citrus fruits. Also, increase starches and other complex carbohydrates by eating six or more daily servings of a combination of breads, cereals, and legumes.

3. Maintain protein intake at moderate levels.

4. Balance food intake and physical activity to maintain appropriate body weight.

5. Alcohol consumption is not recommended. For those who drink alcoholic beverages, limit consumption to the equivalent of 1 ounce of pure alcohol in a single day.

6. Limit total daily intake of salt to 6g or less.

7. Maintain adequate calcium intake.

8. Avoid taking dietary supplements in excess of the RDA (Recommended Dietary Allowance) in any one day.

9. Maintain an adequate intake of fluoride, particularly during the years of primary and secondary tooth formation and growth. Do not overdo this though because fluoride acidity has been discovered to be a source of concern.

RDI (REFERENCE DAILY INTAKE) AND DV (DAILY VALUE)

Reference Daily Intake is a guide to the recommended daily intake of nutrients for healthy adults. The RDI is used to determine the Daily Value of food and is regulated by the Food and Drugs Administration (FDA) in the United States of America and Health Canada in Canada. It is important to note however that the RDI is just a guide to eating healthy. The DI values are based on an average adult's daily requirement of 8700kJ. Your DIs may be higher or lower depending on your energy needs.

ALKALINE AND ACIDIC FOODS

Some foods are considered to be alkaline or acidic depending on their alkali or acid content. Acidic foods include meat, fish, poultry, eggs, grains, diary, and alcohol. Alkaline foods include green vegetables, fruits, peas, beans, lentils, spices, herbs and seasonings, and seeds and nuts.

Experts have made us understand that too much acid in the body is what makes the body prone to diseases; acidity is a major concern these days caused by our food intake of acidic foods, because it causes diseases like arthritis, heart disease, fatigue, cataracts, memory loss, wrinkled skin & premature ageing, cancers, diabetes and other chronic illnesses. Therefore, it is important for us to eat foods that would give our body acid-base balance. What this means in simple terms is to keep the alkaline level and the acidic level balanced. And a good way to determine this is using the PH level.

PH LEVEL

The pH level simply tells you if something is acidic, base (alkaline) or neutral. If the pH level is $0 - 7$, it means the body's acidic content is high, if the pH level is 7 exactly, it means it is neutral. The ideal pH level is between 7.35-7.45. The pH level is usually determined by testing the urine and saliva. But generally, it is important to watch our diet to make sure we are avoiding acidic foods.

FUNCTIONAL MEDICINE

Functional medicine addresses the underlying causes of diseases, using a systems- oriented approach in engaging both patient and practitioner in a systems-oriented approach and engaging both patient and practitioner in a therapeutic partnership. By changing the customary disease-centered focus of medical practitioners to concentrating on the particular patient: functional medicine seeks to address the individual, instead of just an isolated set of symptoms. This new approach to medicine and the treatment of diseases was introduced when it was discovered that not only do we as humans differ in our peculiarities even in our body systems, but also because of the dynamism of diseases and sicknesses visited on us globally, in recent times. It seeks to check the needs of the twenty first century diseases. And one of the discoveries of functional medicine is how diet largely contributes to health issues. Therefore, one of the major features of Functional Medicine focuses on how diet impacts the health and function of a man.

When Functional Medicine consultants observe the part played by nutrition in the development of chronic diseases, they consider multiple body systems, such as the digestive system, the immune system, and the detoxification system, because of the connectedness of those systems and their relation to diet. For instance, because 80% of the immune system is contained in the gastrointestinal system, a person's problems with immunity could be related to faulty digestion instead of a malfunction in the body system.

Functional Medicine upholds that chronic disease is almost always followed by a period of declining health in one or more of the body's systems. Thus, these specialists seek to recognize early the symptoms that indicate primary dysfunction, probably resulting to the disease. Instead of treating symptoms as isolated diseases, Functional Medicine looks at the big picture of health incorporating a patient's genetics, diet, lifestyle and bio-chemical individuality. One of the ways Functional Medicine seeks to address declining health is to provide the foods and nutrients needed to restore function. This is a cost effective, non-invasive intervention that aims to stop the progression into disease. This is definitely a better way of looking at diseases and helping patients. Sometimes, all one needs to be better is a diet change and not necessarily all the time, energy and money hospital treatment requires.

HOW TO READ FOOD LABELS

One of the problems with diet and health is the inability of people to read food labels. But it is as important as every other aspect of dieting because you might be ready to watch what you take in but if you buy packaged foods that are harmful to the body, then the purpose has been defeated. But not to worry, reading food labels is easier than you think even though they can be tricky; all you have to be is observant and interested. Here are some of the things you need to check.

- Make sure you check for calories per serving. This will give you an idea of how much calories you are taking by your number of servings. This way, you will be able to monitor your calories intake.
- Pay attention to the information at the top of the label. This information will inform you on the size of a single serving and the total number of servings for every package.
- Also check the nutritional information panel to know how to choose foods with less saturated fat, added sugars or fiber and so on. Sometimes at the front page, they can add certain nutrients they know would attract you but make sure you check the actual quantity of such nutrient in the nutritional information panel.
- The percentage Daily Value is used to consider the nutrients in one serving that is required for an adult. And the DV depends on individual needs based on age, gender and some other factors. If you want to consume less of a nutrient, go for foods with less than 5% DV and if you want to take in more of a nutrient, go for about 20% DV.
- Remember to decrease your consumption of saturated fats, Trans fat and sodium and at the same time increase your consumption of other nutrients you need such as protein, calcium, dietary fiber, vitamins and all others.

Chapter Three

Overweight and Obesity

Overweight or the chronic obesity refers to body weight that's greater than what is considered healthy for a certain height. The most useful measure of overweight and obesity is body mass index (BMI). Being overweight is common especially where food supplies are plentiful and lifestyles are sedentary. In some countries, up to 65% of the adult population is considered either overweight or obese, and this percentage has increased over the last four decades. Excess weight has also reached epidemic proportions globally, with more than 1 billion adults being either overweight or obese in 2003. By 2013, it had increased to more than 2 billion. And right now, it has almost doubled; weight gain has been recorded increasingly in all age groups because the diets keep getting unhealthier. People keep getting too busy to prepare a proper healthy home cooked meal and they resort to snacks and junk food, which does nothing but worsen their case.

Being overweight is generally caused by the intake of more calories (by eating) than are expended by the body (by exercise and everyday living). Factors that may contribute to this imbalance include: alcoholism, eating disorders (such as binge eating, genetic predisposition hormonal imbalances (e.g. hypothyroidism), insufficient or poor-quality sleep, limited physical exercise and sedentary lifestyle, poor nutrition, metabolic disorders, which could be caused by repeated attempts to lose weight by weight cycling, overeating, psychotropic medication (e.g. olanzapine), incessant smoking and other stimulant withdrawal stress. It could also be caused by some sicknesses. For instance, people who have insulin dependent diabetes and chronically overdose insulin may gain weight, while people who already are overweight may develop insulin tolerance, and in the long run type II diabetes.

CAUSES OF OVERWEIGHT

Sedentary Lifestyle

A lot of people do not live actively. Nothing wrong with watching a bit of TV but spending hours in front of the "Idiot Box", Computers etc. can cause serious lethargy, so engaging in a regular exercise & sport routine becomes a burden and then starts the road that may lead to being overweight and obesity riddled with health problems such as Diabetes, High Blood pressure and so on. For People who are deskbound, a simple solution is to stretch the muscles whilst sitting, Flex their legs, stretch their triceps, the torso and so many more simple exercises.

Lack of Energy Balance

The total amount of food that our body needs depends on age, sex, body size, level of physical activity and whether one is pregnant or breastfeeding. Our body converts the protein, fat and carbohydrate in food to energy. Fat is the most concerted basis of energy. Usually, the energy used to maintain fundamental body processes and the energy taken to digest and engage food are not sufficient to burn the energy that we take in daily. Healthy eating and physical activity are imperative for a healthy energetic life. To maintain a healthy weight, therefore, our energy in and out although do not have to be exactly balanced every day. But it needs to be balanced over time because that is what helps us maintain a healthy weight. Maintaining our weight means balancing the energy going into our body as food and drink and the energy being used for growth and repair, for physical activity, and to keep our bodily functions working. An excess energy intake, even a small amount over a long period, will cause weight gain. Children and adolescents need enough nutritious food to grow and develop normally. Older people need to keep physically active and eat nutritious foods to help maintain muscle strength and a healthy weight.

Genes

Genes have also been severally accused as a major cause of excess weight gain and obesity. Although, many have argued that it all boils down to diet and an active lifestyle, genes do have a major role to play in obesity. Obesity has a strong genetic component. Offspring of obese parents are much more likely to become obese than offspring of lean parents. Sure, genetics may play a part but it's also up to the individual. You basically have to strive to "*BREAK THE PATTERN*". It's surely not easy but definitely not impossible.

Parents play an integral part in imparting the correct lifestyle to their kids especially when children are at an impressionable age. Sedentary parents most times have Sedentary children, whereas active parents help motivate their children in so many ways concerning eating habits, sports activities etc. Not to say that being overweight or obese is completely programmed because our genes are not set in stone contrary to popular belief, although there are strong indications that our genetic components do affect our ability to gain weight, but really, the signals we send our genes have a major effect on which genes are expressed and which are not.

Overeating

These highly engineered junk foods create powerful stimulation of the reward centers in our brains. This is the same stimulation people get from abuse of alcohol and other stimulants. The fact is that junk foods can cause full-blown addiction in susceptible individuals. People lose control over their eating behavior, in the same way as alcoholics lose control over their drinking behavior. Addiction is a complex issue with an organic foundation that can be very challenging to rise above. When you become addicted to something, you practically lose your freedom to choose not to, the 'enjoyment' you get from that particular thing begins to make the choice for you. And some people get addicted to food as a way of escape from something they are dealing with and before they know it, they have added too much weight.

Social Environment

Social environment as defined by encompass the immediate physical surroundings, social relationships, and cultural milieus within which defined groups of people function and interact. Our environment doesn't support healthy lifestyle habits; in fact, it encourages obesity. Lack of access to healthy food, promoting unhealthy foods, fast foods, parental negligence, work schedule all culminate to stop us from inculcating a healthy lifestyle.

Health Conditions

Some hormonal complications could bring about overweight and obesity, they include, underactive thyroid (hypothyroidism), Cushing's syndrome, and polycystic ovarian syndrome (PCOS). Underactive thyroid is a disorder in which the thyroid gland does not produce ample thyroid hormone. Lack of thyroid hormone will decelerate your metabolism and result to weight gain. You will also feel tired and weak. Cushing's syndrome is a condition in which the body's adrenal glands make too much of the hormone cortisol. Cushing's syndrome also can happen if a person takes high amount of some drugs, such as prednisone, for long periods. People who have Cushing's syndrome gain weight, have upper-body obesity, a rounded face, fat around the neck, and thin arms and legs. PCOS on the other hand, is a condition that affects about 5–10 percent of women of childbearing age. Women who have PCOS often are obese, have excess hair growth, and have reproductive problems and other health issues. These problems are caused by high levels of hormones called androgens.

Inadequate Sleep

Not getting enough sleep doesn't just make you tired. It also makes you fat, according to scientists. In a study, participants who slept for five hours each night gained two pounds in weight over a week because they snacked more. They consumed more calories in the form of after-dinner snacks than in any other meal. But when they shifted to adequate sleep patterns they reduced their consumption of fat and carbohydrate and shed the pounds. What happens is when people stay awake; they are most likely to resort to after dinner and late snacks to while away time or just to get over their sleeplessness. Also, most of the weight loss actions in the body occur during sleep, when people do not sleep well, they deprive the body the opportunity of acting on all the plans of weight loss that has been going on all day. So, lack of sleep is not exactly what causes weight gain but what goes on as a result of lack of sleep.

Even though there are records of health related cases and other causes of overweight and obesity, it is clear that they are about ten percent of the statistics and ninety percent other cases are nutrition related or caused by a sedentary life. Adding weight has always been easier than losing it, hence the challenge most overweight people face. They find it very challenging changing their diet and embracing something new. And others begin it but find it hard sticking to the decision they have made. Therefore, it takes not just treatment but also motivation to lose weight.

SYMPTOMS

The basic symptom of obesity is an above normal body weight. It would naturally result in your clothes feeling tight and discovering you need a larger size, the scale showing that you've gained weight, having extra fat around the waist and generally, a higher than normal body mass index and waist circumference. However if you are obese, you may also experience:

- Trouble sleeping.
- Sleep apnea. This is a condition in which breathing is irregular and periodically stops during sleep.
- Shortness of breath.
- Varicose veins.
- Skin problems caused by moisture that accumulates in the folds of your skin.
- Gallstones.
- Osteoarthritis in weight-bearing joints, especially the knees, etc.

TREATMENT

As mentioned earlier, overweight and obesity is very challenging to treat because medical treatment can only do little, the real treatment is determination and motivation to change lifestyle and it has to be consistent because the weight was not gained in a day and so cannot be gone in a day. It did take a while to gain the weight even though it happened unnoticed and it was an easy life but with losing weight, comes difficult and uncomfortable changes. So, there has to be genuine willingness. Some ways where by overweight and obesity can be treated include;

A modified diet

A reasonable weight loss goal is 1 to 2 pounds per week. This can usually be achieved by eating 500 to 1,000 fewer calories each day. Whether you concentrate on eating less fat or fewer carbohydrates is up to you. Fats have more than twice as many calories per ounce than carbohydrates or protein. If you cut out carbohydrates, you still need to limit fat intake. Choose healthy fats, such as monounsaturated and polyunsaturated oils. A healthy eating plan would give your body the nutrients it needs every day. It has enough calories for good health, but not so many that you gain weight. Following the healthy diet religiously will lower your risk for heart disease and other conditions. Some healthy foods include:

- Fat-free and low-fat dairy products, such as low-fat yogurt, cheese, and milk.
- Fresh Fruits
- Whole-grain foods, such as whole-wheat bread, oatmeal, and brown rice. Vegetables, which can be fresh, canned (without salt)
- Protein foods, such as lean meat, fish, poultry without skin, beans, and peas.

Regular Exercise

To successfully drop weight, most people need to do mildly concentrated exercise for 60 minutes most days of the week. But people vary in the amount of physical activity they need to control their weight. Many people can maintain their weight by doing 150 to 300 minutes of mildly concentrated activity per week, such as brisk walking. People who want to lose a large amount of weight might be required to do more than 300 minutes of mildly concentrated activity per week. This also may be true for people who want to keep off weight that they have lost. You do not have to do the activity all at once. You can break it up into short periods of at least 10 minutes each. Also, include additional motion during the day. Take the stairs and get up often from your desk or sofa, walk instead of using the car to get down the block, go to a park and just enjoy the scenery walking, practice intentional stand instead of siting sometimes, do house chores – get the mower out and mow, do something vigorous and sweaty.

Be Realistic

It is true you want to lose that weight and feel better about yourself but it did not take you a day to gain and so it would not take you a day to lose it. What you have as fat accumulated over the years, so give yourself a break. Do not expect to lose 5 pounds a week, you would pressurize yourself and will likely give up more easily. Understand that little drops of water do make an ocean and take it one day at a time. The danger of losing weight too fast is that you would likely gain it back again, so it is better if it is permanent and you can get that by exercises and changing your diet not by some short cut method that you would not have to go through any challenge.

NOW BE CAREFUL OF THOSE DIET PILLS....

Diet pills can be prescribed, especially in the case of obesity to augment the healthy lifestyle already practiced by the individual. Some people also settle for non-prescribed diet pills. Over-the-counter diet pills often contain ingredients that can increase heart rate and blood pressure. It is not clear how effective they are in producing weight loss that can be maintained over time. But it has been discovered over time that most of the people that rely on pills, whether prescribed or self-medicated, regain their weight after use, so they are highly unreliable. Doctors who prescribe it always combine it with calorie-free diet. Also, they usually have side effects in the long run. Therefore, if you are taking pills and you want long-lasting results, make sure it is the right dosage or better still doctor's orders and make sure it is augmented with the right lifestyle of healthy eating plan and exercises. In addition, make sure you go to the right doctor (not your family doctor) who understands weight management and is also a nutritionist.

From the points stated above, losing weight still all boils down to food and staying active. The most effective therefore is changing lifestyle and accepting the changes as a new way of life, instead of as a death sentence. If you embrace it willingly, it is only a matter of time before you get used to it. You would be amazed what our body can adapt to, if we just accept it in our mind! The process might take longer but it would definitely come to be rewarding in the long run.

COMMON MYTHS ABOUT WEIGHT LOSS

A lot of people have being fed with myths about weight loss and they are quickly disillusioned that they believed the wrong thing. The reason for this is not far-fetched, people are so eager to lose weight that they believe everything they hear hook, line and sinker. But luckily, we have found out some of these myths and you are about to find out how true some of the supposed facts you have being fed with are;

All calories are the same

Although all calories have the same energy content, but they most definitely do not have the same effect on your weight or weight loss process. Calories actually go through different metabolism process in the body depending on the food source. For instance, you cannot compare fat, carbs and protein calories, they are different and some are more infilling than others. The calories from fruits are very filling and preferable to those from carbs. Furthermore, substituting carbs and fat with protein can help enhance the body's metabolism, decrease appetite and cravings, at the same time boosting the function of some weight-regulating hormones.

You need to skip meals to lose weight

This is one of the most popular weight loss myths and many people have eaten into it, whereas it is very untrue. Skipping meals does not help reduce weight, as a matter of fact, it does just the opposite. Skipping meals increase your hunger and cravings for food so much that when you finally eat, you take in more portion than required and that harms your weight loss process. Also, skipping meals affects the metabolism and makes it difficult to lose weight because the body will try to overcompensate for what it lost.

Snacking is a total bad idea

You do not have to starve to lose weight. That is one thing you need to understand, so you are free to do away with the belief that after meals snacks is bad. No, not always. Experts actually recommend eating about five smaller meals, instead of larger portions of three meals. When you are hungry and you feel like eating after meals would make you gain weight, actually, what is likely to happen is that you would over eat or binge later. The only way you can help the situation is to make sure you nibble on healthy snacks like nuts and fruits, instead of a burger.

To lose weight, you must avoid fats and carbs

This is not necessarily true. Carbohydrate and fats are actually essential nutrients for our body, so the advice to avoid them is counterproductive. It is a scientific fact that low-carbs diet actually helps with weight loss. What you should avoid is refined carbs like sugar but carbs in general as far as they are low and taken with high amount of protein actually enhance weight loss. Fats also are of different types and there are good fats. Saturated fats found in foods like meat, butter, milk and so on are what should be avoided but unsaturated fats gotten from vegetables and nuts are very healthy. Likewise omega 3-fats oil, gotten from fish are also very good, especially as regards the heart.

Genetics and weight loss

A lot of people and even some nutritionists actually debunk the fact that genetics affect weight loss. But the truth is that it does, and we need to recognize that fact so as not to put ourselves or others under undue pressure. Now, this is not to say it is completely impossible to lose weight, no, it is still possible. But the road is tougher for some people and we need to acknowledge it. Due to some biological factors, some people have slower metabolic rate which causes fats to burn faster and for some, it comes easily.

Diet Pills help you lose weight

All those supplements and diet pills are really not so beneficial but they are actually counterproductive. Not only do they not help the body as most of them have negative side effects, but they are also not permanent. About 80% percent of the time, the subject gains the weight back and in a more dramatic way. If you want to lose weight, then just embrace a healthy lifestyle, it is healthier and more permanent way of losing weight.

Eating breakfast is necessary

This is also a myth as experts have found that eating or skipping breakfast does not have any effect on weight loss. According to Authority Nutrition, a study was recently carried out on 309 men and women to determine how breakfast affects weight loss. They pursued the same lifestyle habits but that of the breakfast. And after a period of four months, it was discovered that eating or skipping breakfast had no effect whatsoever on weight loss. The trick is to eat when you are hungry and stop when you become satisfied. Do not overstuff yourself as well, make sure you eat moderately anytime you eat.

It's quite simple – Yes Breakfast can give you more energy, so if you wake up with hunger pangs – EAT & ENJOY THE EVENT and if you don't, it's ok, don't clobber yourself over it!

Eating and exercising consistently will prevent weight gain

While this is true in the general scheme of things, we need to understand that it is important to be flexible with our lifestyle habits, as we age. This is because as we age, our metabolism become slower and would not be able to burn fat as it did when we were younger. So there are times when we would need to eat less and exercise more and vice versa. Just make sure to stay healthy in whatever method you employ.

"Diet" foods help with weight loss

We need to know that this "diet" foods industry is large and a lot of times, they beautify their marketing strategy to attract people. Some of these foods are not as fat-free, gluten-free or sugar-free as they like to make us believe. The truth is many at times, if it is a processed food, then it is likely unhealthy unlike what we see on their packages.

Thin is healthy while fat is unhealthy

This is one of the biggest myths ever because you can be thin and unhealthy and you can be fat and healthy. There are people who are thin but have chronic diseases and people who are overweight but are biologically healthy. Although fats are associated with a lot of other diseases, but it depends on where the fat is stored. If the fats escape the abdomen and the organs of the body, then you are relatively safe, fats stored under the skin, the subcutaneous fat, is more of a cosmetic problem. Now this is not to say that you should be comfortable being overweight, you still need to shed it, but this is more like a call to thin people to make sure they are healthy by also watching their diet and adequate exercising.

Losing weight is a straight road

No, this is not true. There are days when you would add weight even though you are in the process of losing weight and it does not have to mean something is wrong with the process. It could just mean that you are holding more food in your system or your body contains more water at that point in time. As far the days you add weight is not more than when you lose it, then you are good to go.

UNDERWEIGHT

I know a lot of us think being overweight is the only problem there is. But it is also a problem if we are underweight and it should be taken with as much seriousness as we do overweight. Underweight is simply defined as having a weight that is less than normal, required or healthy. For one to be considered underweight, that means the person's body mass index must be less than 18.5 or 15 to 20% below the normal weight for their age and height. We are experiencing more cases of underweight not really because of constant preaching to lose weight and avoid obesity but also because society has embraced or linked beauty to slim people. So a lot of women are facing pressure to lose weight and this pressure makes them over do it, leading to underweight. Although the percentage of people who are underweight are still relatively low compared to those who are overweight but that does not reduce the severity of the situation as well. This is because being underweight brings with it cases like malnutrition, physical defects, weak immune system – leaving them open to diseases, mental diseases and even death. Being underweight really presents a risk, leading to health difficulties which are more challenging to cure.

CAUSES OF UNDERWEIGHT

Some of the causes of underweight include the following;

Physical Causes

Physical causes like sickness could be at the root of being underweight. Sometimes, when someone is underweight, it just goes to show that there are underlying issues and most of the underlying issues are sicknesses or diseases that are accompanied with weight loss. Some of these diseases include; diabetes, intestinal parasite, Hyperthyroidism, cancer, inflammatory bowel disease and others. All these diseases can cause one to be underweight and so; it is advisable to go for check up to determine the particular cause before it degenerates into something more serious.

Hereditary

There are quite a number of people who are underweight as a result of their genes. If one or both of one's parents are underweight or mildly underweight, then it could likely rub off on that person. Some people have a naturally faster metabolism than others and their body reacts to food differently from others. And for some, it could be that they do not have as many fat cells and consequently their body has less space to store fat.

Environmental and Social Factors

Environmental factors like poverty, famine, drought or even economic recession causes underweight in some societies. Poverty is a wide range cause of underweight. A lot of people, especially in underdeveloped and developing countries live on less than a dollar standard of living. And due to this, they feed poorly. This could leave a lot of people, especially children, malnourished. Also closely related to this, is famine and drought and other factors that would discourage food production, resulting in malnourishment and ultimately, underweight situations.

Eating Habits

Your eating habits could also contribute to massive weight loss. If you are eating irregularly, skipping meals, constant fasting; then you are at a risk of being underweight. Apart from that, even eating at odd hours could upset your body system and metabolism and prevent the adequate amount of fat needed for the body.

Depression

Depression could come as a result of anything and it could be just as a result of stress. If a person is depressed, there is a high chance the person would become underweight. This is due to the fact that a lot of depressed people will either become emotional eaters or they completely lose appetite because of how low they feel psychologically. In some extreme cases, some may want to punish their body for one reason or the other. Either way, if they are not eating properly, they are likely to get underweight.

Excessive Dieting and Exercises

As a result of trying to lose weight, a lot of people overdo it and become underweight instead of having the required weight. Although dieting is beneficial and even encouraged for good health, but everything should be done in moderation. If it excessive, then chances are you would become lethargic and also lose too much weight. Additionally, if you do more exercises than your body needs, chances are that you would lose weight drastically. As much as exercises are preached and really encouraged because of the load of good it does to the body, it can also be overdone and cause problems in the body. So if exercises are overdone, they also result to the problem of underweight.

Medication

Some medication can also make people lose weight, even the prescribed ones because their side effects could be loss of appetite. Pill Abuse also affects the body system, also resulting to weight loss.

SYMPTOMS OF UNDERWEIGHT

The symptoms of extreme weight loss are weakness, feeling lethargic, fatigue, loss of appetite, and increase in illnesses and disease due to the weak immune system. Weight loss that is as a result of an underlying disease would likely be accompanied with other symptoms. But either way, make sure you visit a medical practitioner to be sure what exactly is wrong.

TREATMENT

Being underweight is not a disease, so the treatment does not really involve expert care, except for cases where it is a symptom of a more serious disease. The treatment of a normal case of underweight just like that of overweight involves changing lifestyle. Some of the ways include;

Diet

Underweight people would have to increase their weight through change of dieting. Instead of avoiding calories, they would be required to include it in their meals. But of course, everything would still have to be done with extreme care and in moderation. Calorie-dense meals like rice, dried fruits, butter, cheese, and nuts should be encouraged. Also good sources of protein and of course minerals and vitamins are also highly recommended. Such a person would have to avoid skipping meals and maybe even fasting till there is considerable weight gain.

Exercises

Yes, exercises are also necessary for weight gain. Some exercises like weight lifting encourages weight gain. Although exercises are catabolic, resulting in reduction of the body mass, however, weight gain can occur through anabolic overcompensation. What happens is that the body overcompensates through muscle hypertrophy when there is too much catabolism going on and that would bring about weight gain. So you could visit the gym and let the trainer know you are in on your weight gain process, so you would be put through some exercise routines that would encourage weight gain.

Appetite Boosts

You could also take the right supplements which would increase your appetite; especially if your case is lack of appetite. You should to consult a good nutritionist or your doctor who can give you the right advise. So be sure to consult your doctor before trying them.

From the foregoing, we can see that underweight is just as serious as overweight. So in our bid to lose weight, let us not overdo it and always remember *"MODERATION IS THE KEY"*

BMI

BMI, the acronym for Body Mass Index is a calculation used to determine one's weight. The BMI is an attempt to quantify the amount of tissue mass (muscle, fat, and bone) in an individual, and then categorize that person as underweight, normal weight, overweight, or obese based on that value. It is calculated by dividing ones weight in kilograms by the square of one's height in meters. The accepted unit therefore is expressed in units of kg/m2. But it could be calculated with pounds and feet, in that instance, a conversion would be required. The standard BMI ranges are underweight: under 18.5, normal weight: 18.5 to 25, overweight: 25 to 30, obese: over 30.

BMI FORMULA – (body weight in kg) / (body height in m) 2. For instance if a person has a height of 1.65m and a body weight of 60kg, we would multiply the height by itself. That is, 1.65 * 1.65 = 2.7225. Then divide the result by the weight. That is, 60/2.7225 = 22. This particular person's BMI is 22, which is a healthy BMI.

Chapter Four

Mind and Body Connection

The connection of the mind and body just explains how our mind affects our body and vice versa. If we are happy and in a good mood, our body too would be in form and in good health. So also, if our body is in good health, our minds would be at alert. However, on the other hand, if we are sad, moody or depressed, it automatically affects our body. That is the reason why people who are stressed or depressed are usually faced with different kinds of health issues that affects them. In the context of health and nutrition, times without number, people with stress feel really unhappy with themselves, and even though they don't mean to, cause harm to their body by binge and emotional eating. If we want to live in good health, then we have to try to live positively. Life will always throw us a curve ball but it is how we respond to it that would determine the state of our health.

EMOTIONAL EATING

Emotional eating has to do with eating to manage stress. It is a way people react to stress by eating, which is why some medical practitioners call it, 'stress eating.' Among other factors, researchers have linked weight gain to stress, and according to an American Psychological Association survey, 75% of adults reported experiencing moderate to high levels of stress, and it has gotten worse today not better. Eating when we are stressed or when we are trying to juggle too many activities in such limited time or unpleasant emotions not only affects what we eat, but how we digest what we eat.

At the initial stage, stress can shut down appetite. A structure in the brain called the hypothalamus produces corticotrophin-releasing hormone, which suppresses appetite. However, when it starts getting advanced and in some cases moving towards depression, the adrenal glands discharge an additional hormone called cortisol, and cortisol increases appetite and may also increase motivation in general, including the motivation to eat. The problem with emotional eating, unlike mindful eating is that they are usually foods with high calories. This is probably because at that point, the main thing one wants is something that would make one feel good, and that is why they are called, 'comfort food.' The foods that emotional eaters crave are often referred to as comfort foods, like ice cream, cookies, chocolate, chips, French fries, and pizza. About forty percent of people tend to eat more when stressed, while about forty percent eat less and twenty percent experience no change in the amount of food they eat when exposed to stress.

On the flip side, stress even when you are not exactly eating much can still resort to weight gain. Our body system responds to even outside stimuli, which is why we feel the responses to fear, sadness or just rush. When we are stressed, our bodies' natural inclination also would be to respond to that situation and one of such responses is the shutdown of our digestive system. The message we are practically passing to it is not to digest at that particular time because an emergency is going on. and so, even if we are eating so little at this point, the body would likely not digest, causing it to be stored as fat. To the body, these stimuli, while not as dramatic or intense as being in terrifying, they are still being regarded as "emergency". Hence, we are likely to experience the digestive symptoms such as heartburn, a feeling of food just sitting in your stomach, bloating, belching, and overall stomach pain. The nutritional value of even the healthiest meal is diminished because the digestive system isn't functioning optimally to absorb the nutrients.

The warning sign that one has the tendency to emotionally eat is when you discover you resort to food when you are angry, stressed, sad, hurt, restless, lonely, bored and all kinds of emotions. And most times, emotional eaters do not go for a healthy meal, most times, they crave something sweet and resort to snacks or general junk food.

Can it be treated? Yes, it can and needs to be treated before it complicates to obesity or other sicknesses that are as a result of overweight. Some of the steps to take to treat emotional eating include;

Eat when you are Hungry: Most emotional eaters have discovered their tendency to overeat, so they starve themselves and avoid eating when they are hungry. But this has a counter effect because what happens at the end is that they would eat more than is needed when they do finally eat. As a matter of fact, starving to lose weight has been discouraged numerous times because you do not end up achieving what you have set to achieve. Not only would you overcompensate later by eating too much, but your body would also react harshly by storing up fat to survive the starvation. So when you are hungry get something nourishing in a reasonable portion and eat.

Exercises: Regular physical activity tends to dampen the production of stress chemicals, even leading to a decrease in depression, anxiety, and insomnia in addition to decreasing the tendency to engage in emotional eating. Intense exercise increases cortisol levels temporarily, but low-intensity exercise seems to reduce them. According to researchers exercise may possibly decrease some of the negative effects of stress. And on the other hand, exercises actually do make us feel good about ourselves; it refreshes us and would likely lighten our mood.

DON'T HESITATE TO MEDITATE!

Myriad researches have shown that meditation lessens stress, granted much of the research has focused on high blood pressure and heart disease. Engaging in meditation and other relaxation techniques is a powerful way to decrease emotional eating. Meditation may also help people become more mindful of food choices. With practice, a person may be able to pay better attention to the impulse to grab a comfort food and inhibit the impulse.

Therefore, engaging in one or two meditation sessions a day can have lasting beneficial effects on health, even decreasing high blood pressure and heart rate.

Stay Positive: Approach life from an optimistic perspective and don't let bad situations get to you. Understand that bad situations could always happen but you do not have to let them affect you. And if you are faced with uncomfortable and challenging situations, approach your feelings with kindness, and your body will begin to understand that it no longer has to overeat to protect you from your feelings. Also, allow yourself to feel and cultivate the habit of telling yourself it would be alright. By listening to your emotions, you'll discover what it is you truly want, and can create new strategies for deeper satisfaction.

Chapter Five

Sleep

Sleep: Nature's soft nurse – ***Shakespeare***

A lot of people have mixed up the concept of sleep. Most of us seem to think sleep is a luxury we cannot afford to have or that sleep is a way of adding weight. Well, of course, everything done in excess is not good. There is practically nothing good in this world that does not turn problematic if done excessively. So yes, too many hours spent sleeping is equivalent to living a sedentary lifestyle and we have outlined what that can do to the health previously.

However, the benefit is adequate sleep cannot be overemphasized. Sleeping is so important Shakespeare called it "nature's soft nurse". We all know what it means to nurse; it is synonymous with care. Sleep is like giving our body the care it needs after all the usual stress it goes through throughout the day. Our bodies need a well-deserved rest after the day's work and sleeping can accord it that. And contrary to popular belief, you are actually likely to lose more weight if you allow your body the appropriate sleep time it needs than when you do not sleep.

It has been discovered by nutritionists and medical practitioners that people who find it hard to sleep are more prone to weight gain because the hours when you are awake, you are likely to be tempted to feed on foods that are calorie rich. Somebody who is awake is usually not going for the green salads at that time; The foods that would mostly be preferred are sweetened foods that would boost weight gain. Also, although the body is resting during sleep, it is also very active. It is not in a passive stage as initially believed. So the processes that lead to weight loss amidst others are usually carried out in the night. If you have spent your day exercising, eating well-balanced meals and you do not let the body work on the effort you have put in to get you the result you want, you would practically have wasted your time. And apart from weight loss, you would be depriving the body of all the essential metabolic processes that goes on during sleep.

What is sleep?

Sleep is the state of reduced consciousness during which a human or animal rests in a daily rhythm. Encarta dictionary went more elaborate and describes sleep as a state of partial or full unconsciousness in people, and animals, during which voluntary functions are suspended and the body rests and restores itself. We would note that the dominant term in both definitions is rest and in the latter definition, it is pointed out that the body restores itself during sleep.

The state of being awake and that of sleep are all as a result of activities of the brain. There are nerve-signals called neurotransmitters control that control sleep and being awake by activating certain neurons in the brain. Neurons in the brainstem, which connects the brain with the spinal cord, produce neurotransmitters such as serotonin and norepinephrine that keep some parts of the brain active while we are awake. Further neurons at the base of the brain begin signaling when we fall asleep. These neurons seem to switch the signals that keep us awake off. New discovery also submits that a chemical called adenosine develops in our blood while we are awake and brings about drowsiness. This chemical gradually breaks down while we sleep.

Experts have also described sleep into different stages; we have the REMS and the NON REMS. The non REMS are further divided into four stages. We have being told our sleep occurs averagely in periods of about 90 minutes and throughout the 90 minutes, we go through different stages of sleep.

NON REMS SLEEP: As mentioned earlier, it occurs in four phases, phase 1, 2, 3, and 4.

Stage 1 is the period of light or drowsy sleep and can be easily awaken. In this stage, the eyes move slowly and muscle activity slows. Many people also experience a sensation that can be likened to falling, it is the same feeling we experience when we are startled. We also are likely to lose some muscle tone and most conscious awareness of the external environment.

Stage 2 is the period of total sleep and we are now difficult to awake when we reach this phase of sleep. Again, our eye movement stops, brain waves become slower and we experience an occasional burst of rapid brain waves.

Stage 3 is the period of deep, slow wave sleep and we are less responsive to our environment. Our body begins to experience extremely slow brain waves called delta waves, interposed with smaller, faster waves.

Stage 4 is the period of the deepest sleep and we are completely unaware of our environment. There is no eye movement or muscle activity in this phase. People awakened from the stage four usually have a harder time adjusting to the environment for some moments.

REMS (Rapid Eye Movement): In this phase, humans experience rapid eye movement (REM), temporary paralyzed muscles, and unregulated heart rate, breathing and body temperature. This is the phase where most of us have dreams and when awoken, we are likely to remember it. Most people experience three to five intervals of REM sleep every night.

Benefits of Sleep

1. Adequate sleep is very important for the brain. Sleep deprivation leads to impaired memory and makes it difficult for us to concentrate well the next day.

2. Many of the body's cells show improved production and lowered breakdown of proteins during deep sleep.

3. Satisfactory sleep is involved in healing and repair of your heart and blood vessels.

4. Lack of sleep may make neurons become so depleted in energy or so polluted with byproducts of normal cellular processes that they begin to breakdown.

5. Sleep also reduces our feeling of irritation and uplifts our mood. As a matter of fact, scientists have discovered that lack of sleep has been found to cause depression and suicide.

6. Adequate sleep has again being discovered to improve the immune system and keep the body from diseases. A good time spent sleeping has been associated with a reduced risk of cancer and heart diseases.

7. Sleep also supports healthy growth and development. Adequate sleep activates the body to discharge the hormone that stimulates proper growth in children and teens.

8. Sleep helps sustain a healthy equilibrium of the hormones that make us feel hungry (ghrelin) or satisfied (leptin). Inadequate sleep increases the ghrelin and reduces the leptin, thereby making us eat more and resulting to overweight and obesity.

9. Lack of sleep has also caused non-biological problems like tragic accidents due to fatigue and sleepiness.

Now, we might wonder how then do we determine healthy sleep? An average adult needs about 8 hours sleep daily to function. However, it has also been discovered that the hours needed varies. Some people can function with less and others need more. For instance, Albert Einstein slept 12 hours a day and he was one of the most intelligent scientists to ever live. So it cannot be concluded that anyone who sleeps more than 8 hours is over-sleeping or one who sleeps less is suffering from deficiency. Scientist has found a way out and they suggest that deficiency can be determined by the way we feel during the day. If we feel restless, sleepy, drowsy, and irritable during the day, chances are we did not have enough sleep.

Also, the quality of sleep is usually taken into consideration as well. It is not only how far but how well. So if for any reason, we sleep many hours and still feel some of the above symptoms, then it is possible that we did not have quality sleep. And the major factor that militates against sleep apart from stress is our diet. If we do not eat healthy or take in food, like caffeine, that interrupts the neurons in control of sleep, it would affect the quality of our sleep.

INSOMNIA OR SLEEP DISORDER

As important as sleep is and as we have even established above that it is not a waste of time, unfortunately, a lot of people still suffer from lack of sleep or what is called insomnia. Insomnia is simply defined by the Encarta dictionary as the inability to fall asleep or to remain asleep long enough to feel rested, especially when this is a problem that continues over time. As we have also established above, different people need different hours of sleep in order to feel rested, therefore, insomnia is determined by the quality of your sleep and how you feel after sleeping and not necessarily the number of hours you spend sleeping or how quickly you doze off.

There are different categories of insomnia depending on how long it last and how it occurs. The transient insomnia usually last for a few nights, the short-term insomnia last for a few weeks but when it proceeds three to four weeks, then it is chronic insomnia. Also, there is primary insomnia which is characterized by difficulty in falling asleep and constantly waking up during the night, whereas secondary insomnia is usually associated with a symptom of an underlying disease.

CAUSES OF INSOMNIA

Insomnia is caused by a variety of reasons and it varies with individuals. But below are some common causes of sleep disorder or lack of sleep;

Illnesses or Diseases

Illnesses or diseases such as hyperthyroidism, Parkinson's disease, diabetes, lupus, asthma, cancer, and kidney diseases have being associated with insomnia. These diseases have being known to rob people of sleep, so the insomnia could be as a result of some other issues.

Anxiety and Depression

The rate at which stress, anxiety, depression rob people of their sleep cannot be overemphasized. It is usually important to leave the issues of the day outside the bed so as to enjoy proper sleep. If we do not properly manage stress, they have adverse effect on our sleep and general health.

Medications

Some drugs actually have effect on our general body system and affect our sleep pattern. Drugs such as antidepressants, stimulants for ADHD, corticosteroids, thyroid hormone, high blood pressure medications, some contraceptives, cold and flu medications that contain alcohol, pain relievers that contain caffeine (Midol, Excedrin), diuretics, and slimming pills have been known to cause sleep disorder as a side effect.

Menopause and Pregnancy

Many women have experienced loss of their beauty sleep during pregnancy or when they attain menopause as a result of the hormonal changes that their body experiences. Menopausal women experience hot flashes and sweating which can make it difficult to sleep, especially in the initial stage. Also the discomfort associated with pregnancy can make the woman lose sleep.

Lifestyle

Sometimes, the sleep disorder that people experience is as a result of their lifestyle. There are some things that you likely do which trigger loss of sleep. Activities like sleeping in a noisy environment, drinking caffeinated drinks, exercising or eating late, keeping irregular sleep schedule, watching television or active on your computer or phone late at night, can affect your sleep as well.

SYMPTOMS OF INSOMNIA

Symptoms of insomnia include drowsiness, lack of mental alertness and, sluggishness, trouble getting back to sleep after waking up, restlessness, difficulty concentrating during the day, lack of feeling of refreshment after sleeping and so on.

TREATMENT OF INSOMNIA

It is important to go see a medical practitioner especially if you honestly cannot identify why you cannot sleep and symptoms persists. If you figure out it is as a result of stress or lifestyle, then you can just change it but if you cannot figure out the reason or if it is accompanied by other symptoms, then the insomnia is probably as a result of an underlying illness and the only way to treat it would be to treat the primary illness. Nonetheless, below are some ways to treat insomnia;

Lifestyle change

If you discover for any reason that you have gotten into the habit of some of the activities listed above, other things being equal, that is the only problem you have and all you have to do is embrace change. Change all those things that deprive you of good, restive sleep and you are good to go. For instance;

- Avoid stimulating activities late in night. Activities like watching television, handling computers, video games and smart phones or even exercising late at night.
- Avoid eating late into the night. Sometimes, indigestion keeps people awake. Try to eat at least four hours before bed time.
- Do regular exercises as it helps keep your body healthy and also helps you sleep well. However, remember not to do it late at night.
- Avoid alcohol and caffeinated drinks; they tamper with your sleep time.
- Avoid napping during the day and keep regular sleeping schedule. Sometimes when we nap, our body has already had the amount of sleep it needs. So the best way to deal with it is to avoid naps. Additionally, if you keep irregular sleep schedules, you confuse your body clock and it would have a hard time determining when you are supposed to be asleep and awake.
- Keep your room cool, quiet and relaxed. Chances are you would not find much sleep in a noisy room that is also not conducive. So if you want to sleep well, you have to make sure that is also taken care of.
- Eat a balanced diet. You might be wondering why everything has to boil down to diet but the truth is that almost every aspect of our lives is connected to what we put in our mouth. So if you need your beauty sleep, make sure you are eating the right things.

Try to live a positive lifestyle

When you go to bed with so much anxieties, stress and worries, chances are you would not get any sleep. Try to keep the problems of the day in the day and be positive that the next day would be better. But when you spend your time stressing over issues, it would affect your sleep and your health in general. And when you cannot sleep immediately, don't panic, try to relax and meditate on happy things.

Sleeping pills

Sleeping pills can be effective in helping you sleep but a lot of people do not recommend it because it is counterproductive in the long run. Not only do they not give sound, quality sleep, they also have side effects. Additionally, a lot of people come to rely on them and instead of them curing the sleep problem, they just encourage drug abuse. So if at all, sleep supplements would be administered, it is usually advisable to go for simple remedies like lemon balm or chamomile tea and some drugs such as Melatonin and Valerian.

You might need to seek professional help, especially if it is serious. If you find out the insomnia is not responding to all we have listed above; if it is causing problems at work or it is recurrent and nothing seems to be working for it, then that is an indication that you need to go see a medical practitioner.

In the long run, it is better to embrace change for a more effective sleep. As far as it is not a secondary insomnia, which would then need to be treated by treating the root illness, then changing habits and imbibing certain cultures would go a long way in helping. Everybody wants to enjoy beauty sleep because of how beneficial it is and like Shakespeare said, it really is nature's soft nurse, so it is important you get the best quality sleep. Not only for the satisfaction it brings, but also because of the health benefits.

SLEEP APNEA

Sleep apnea is a disorder whereby the victim experiences shortness of breath and breath difficulty in the midst of sleep. It is characterized by breath pauses that can last for few seconds or minutes and can occur for up to thirty times throughout the night. Sleep apnea is not restricted by age or gender; it can occur to people of all ages, even children. In most cases, most people suffering from sleep apnea are unaware they have the disorder, although their sleep is interrupted by frequent shortness of breath. This is probably because when they are awaken, their breathing is restored to normal and they might not remember they were awaken in their sleep because they were not fully awaken when they did or they just forget out rightly. And since there is no routine check or blood test to determine it, it can go for years unchecked. In most cases, it is a sleeping partner that discovers that there is a disorder. And untreated sleep apnea can result to other chronic diseases like heart attack, obesity, high blood pressure, and stroke.

CAUSES

- Sleep apnea usually occurs in people who are overweight. The extra fat tissue they have can thicken the wall of the windpipe, narrowing the windpipe. And when we are sleeping, the throat muscles naturally relax unlike when we are awake that they keep the airways stiff and open so air can flow freely to the lungs.
- Naturally some people have smaller airway size in the throat and mouth area.
- Age could also relax the throat muscles and prevent them from making the airway stiff as expected.

SYMPTOMS

Some of the symptoms include loud and ongoing snoring, tiredness, sore or dry throat upon waking up, headache, sleepiness during the day, sour mood, forgetfulness and sometimes you might notice gasping when you sleep. If you feel any of these, visit a doctor and the medical practitioner would do some tests which could include sleeping over while your sleep is recorded on a video.

TREATMENT

- Some people with sleep apnea might be told to embrace some lifestyle changes especially if the sleep apnea is caused by overweight. You might be asked to simply lose some weight.

- CPAP (Continuous Positive Airway Pressure) is the most common treatment used. It is a machine that consists of a specially fitted mask to cover your mouth and/or nose while you sleep. The machine supplies a continuous flow of air into your nostrils and promotes open airway for easy breathing.
- Dental devices like a mouthpiece are also used to treat sleep apnea. The device will be used to keep the airways open for free and easy flow of air to the lungs.

On the final analysis, sleep is a very important lifestyle to imbibe in keeping our body nourished and far from diseases. Sleep is no longer a waste of time as formerly believed. It is also a necessary part of our body process. So if we find anything obstructing our sleep, before it degenerates into something more serious, it would do us a world of good to try to do something about it.

Chapter Six

Super Foods

You don't have to eat less, you just have to eat right. - **Unknown**

We have a lot of meals that people disregard but these foods are exactly what we need to get us where we want health-wise. These foods are unlike our everyday wants but they would go a long way in keeping us from all the diseases plaguing the world today. The dictionary defines super food as "a nutrient- rich food considered to be especially beneficial for health and well-being." They contain sparse calories and are full of nutrients which are beneficial to the body and those are the kind of meals we should be pursuing. Earlier, it was established that we should be kind to ourselves and feed our body what it needs and not necessarily or not always what it wants. An editorial published in the American Journal of Clinical Nutrition (2007) noted in response to this study - we are spending millions to find drugs that can impact our production of hormones such as insulin, when there might already be a simple dietary strategy. The editorial concluded by saying, "The results of the present study emphasize the age old wisdom to use food as medicine. One of the major misconceptions that have plagued healthy living is that healthy foods are boring. Surprisingly enough, most of these foods are interesting and delicious. Once you get over your prejudice, you would come to love them. Some of them include;

FRUITS

1. Spirulina: Spirulina is a cyanobacteria often referred to as blue-green algae, that is valued as a rich source of protein, containing vitamins, minerals, essential fatty acids, and antioxidants. It grows in both fresh and salt water. Spirulina is a source for amino acids, iron, chlorophyll, phosphorus, zinc and most other vitamins.
   - 'Spirulina is a good detoxifier and helps remove toxins from the body.
   - Spirulina can lower LDL "bad" cholesterol and Triglyceride levels, while increasing the HDL "good" cholesterol.
   - It is also known to boost the immune system.
   - It helps the body fight against oral cancer and also reduce blood pressure.
   - It can also help to burn fat faster during exercise.

2. Apples: Studies have shown that an apple everyday would keep you away from the doctor. Apple is a sweet, pomaceous fruit belonging to the rose family. It is a food rich in fiber, vitamin C and numerous antioxidants.
   - Apples have been said to also have many benefits on the human body. Recent research has shown that apple polyphenols can help avert spikes in blood sugar through a variety of mechanisms.
   - Apples can significantly lower many of our blood fats.
   - Apples are particularly important in prevention of heart disease through healthy regulation of blood fat levels.
   - Apples are very satisfying and good for snacks, especially when you are hungry between meals.
   - The antioxidants in apples help repair oxidation damage that happens during normal cell activity.

3. Grapes: Grape is a green or purple round or oval berry with sweet juicy flesh. Grapes can be eaten in various ways including; wine, fruit salad, jelly, and raisin or just as a fruit. It is a good source of vitamin

A, vitamin B, vitamin C, magnesium, potassium, iron, dietary fiber, resveratrol, flavonols, carotenoids, phenolic acids and many more nutrients.

- Grapes help in treating constipation, indigestion, fatigue and kidney disorders.
- They lower the risk of excessive and unwanted inflammation in the body.
- They lower risk of heart disease, diabetes, cancer and other conditions.
- Grapes have been said to decrease mortality rates and improve longevity.
- Grapes also may prevent the feared middle-aged increase in weight and even help you to shed the pound.

4. Watermelon: Delicious & Juicy Watermelon is a large sprawling annual plant rich in lycopene, pantothenic acid, copper, biotin, potassium, vitamin A (in the form of carotenoids), vitamin B1, vitamin B6, and magnesium.

- Watermelons allow blood to flow more freely and create a drop in blood pressure.
- It is important for optimal eye health and boosts immunity by enhancing the infection-fighting actions of white blood cells called lymphocytes.
- It helps the body to avoid over-accumulation of body fat.
- It nourishes the body for a healthy skin.

5. Strawberries: Strawberries are very delicious, highly nutritious, and are low in both carbs and calories. They are rich in potassium, vitamin C, vitamin K, manganese, iron, and many other nutrients and have been listed by researchers as one of the best antioxidants among popular foods in the world.

- It is related with the reduction of blood sugar levels.
- They contain powerful antioxidants and are thought to protect against inflammation, cancer and heart disease.

- They are of great value to the cardiovascular system by preventing cardiovascular diseases.
- Strawberries have been used to treat digestive ailments, teeth whitening and skin irritations.

VEGETABLES

6. Broccoli: It is an edible green plant in the cabbage family whose large flowering head is eaten as a vegetable. It is another amazing dish that can keep your body nourished. It contains dietary fiber, pantothenic acid, vitamin B6, vitamin E, manganese, phosphorus, choline, vitamin B1, vitamin A (in the form of carotenoids), potassium, and copper. Some of the benefits include;
    - It lowers cholesterol level when cooked by steaming.
    - Kaempferol found in broccoli helps lessen the impact of allergy-related substances on our body.
    - Broccoli is a good detoxification agent; helps remove toxins from the body.
    - Broccoli, like all cruciferous vegetables, has been associated with a lower risk of cancer; especially lung and colon cancer.

7. Asparagus: Asparagus is a spring vegetable, a flowering perennial plant species in the genus Asparagus. They're considered to be one of the delicacies of the vegetable world. They are low in both carbs and calories and rich in fiber, folate, vitamins A, vitamins C, vitamins E, vitamins K, and chromium.
    - Asparagus is anti-inflammatory because it is a source of anti-inflammatory nutrients like quercetin and rutin and more.
    - It enhances the ability of insulin to transport glucose from the bloodstream into cells.
    - It decreases the risk of obesity, diabetes and heart diseases.
    - Asparagus contain folate and folate is good during pregnancy, for children and adolescents to aid growth.

8. Garlic: Garlic is a bulb or clove with a pungent odor and flavor. It is a species in the onion genus, Allium. It specially contains a sulfur compound called Allicin which is very medicinal.

    - Garlic may improve iron metabolism because it contains a protein called ferroportin. Ferroportin moves around the cell membrane, and it forms a passageway that allows stored iron to leave the cells and become available where it is needed.
    - Garlic is known to boost immune function and help fight the common cold, the world's most common infectious disease.
    - Garlic can cause major reductions in blood pressure, thereby reducing the risk of heart diseases and cardiac arrest.
    - It may also control the amount of fat cells that get formed in our system.
    - Garlic contains antioxidants that may help prevent Alzheimer's disease and Dementia.

9. Carrots: Carrot are very good source of carotene antioxidants, fiber, and a lot of other nutrients. Although the orange colored ones are the most popular ones, there are other colors, including white, yellow, red, or purple.

    - Carrots decrease the threat of lung cancer, breast cancer and colon cancer.
    - They protect against cardiovascular disease (CVD).
    - Carrots contain vitamin A, which when broken down can be turned to rhodopsin, a purple pigment that improves vision.
    - Vitamin A and antioxidants in carrots help protect the skin from sun damage.

It is known to increase nutrient absorption, lower risk of allergy, and lower risk of colon cancer. They improve blood pressure, improve blood sugar regulation, and control of blood fat levels.

10. Onions: Onion, also known as common onion or bulb onion is a round or oval edible bulb vegetable with hard pungent flesh in

concentric layers beneath a papery brown skin. They contain a number of bioactive compounds known to be beneficial to the body system. They are loaded with vitamin B, vitamin C, biotin, manganese, copper, potassium, folate and many more.

- Onions lower the risk of some types of cancer, particularly, colorectal, laryngeal, and ovarian cancer.
- They are good for reducing inflammation and healing infections.
- They serve as good support for bones and connective tissues, and are especially beneficial to women of menopausal age who are experiencing loss of bone density.
- Raw onion lowers the production of bad cholesterol (LDL).
- Onions also assist in regulating blood sugar.

11. Potatoes: Potato is a round and starchy tuber from the scientific family of perennial nightshade Solanum tuberosum L, cooked in a variety of ways. They are rich in vitamin B3, vitamin B6, vitamin C, iron, potassium, fiber, pantothenic acid among others.

- Potatoes contain vitamin B6, which is essential for the development of new cells in the body.
- Potato, through vitamin B6, helps relax the body for good sleep and also helps the body respond to stress.
- It is important for normal brain cells function.
- And also, it is beneficial for cardiovascular protection.

12. Celery: Celery is a long crisp, flattish leaf stalk of a cultivated marshland plant variety in the family Apiaceae. Celery contains phenols, pantothenic acid, vitamin A, vitamin B2, vitamin B6, vitamin K, folate, molybdenum, copper, magnesium and a host of others.

- The minerals in celery, especially magnesium, and the vital oil in it, calm the nervous system.
- Celery contains pectin-based polysaccharides that can provide the stomach with aids and protect the whole digestive tract. It also assists in digestion. Celery contains minimal calories and therefore serves as a good alternative food for watching the weight.

- It regulates the alkaline balance of the body system, reducing issues like acidity.

SPICES

13. Ginger: Ginger is the hot, aromatic, pungent, and spicy edible stem rhizome of an Asian plant. Ginger is largely encouraged as one of the healthiest foods in the world because of its vast benefits. It contains vitamin B6, vitamin C, iron, magnesium, dietary fiber, potassium and many more.
    - Ginger has a long history of relieving digestive problems such as nausea, loss of appetite, motion sickness and pain.
    - It is good for arthritis patients as it helps them relieve pain from muscular swelling and reduces swelling,
    - Ginger decreases the risk of obesity, diabetes, heart disease and overall mortality.
    - It provides protection against colorectal cancer.
    - Ginger nourishes the body by promoting a healthy complexion and hair, and increasing energy.

14. Basils: Basil, also known as Saint Joseph's Wort, is a culinary herb with aromatic leaves belongs to the family Lamiaceae. It has also been termed "the king of herbs" or "royal herb." Basil is a source of vitamin A, vitamin C, vitamin K, manganese, omega 3-fats, copper, folate, iron, calcium and other nutrients.
    - Orientin and vicenin, the two water-soluble flavonoids found in basil, protect cell structures as well as chromosomes from radiation and oxygen-based damage.
    - Basil is found to be useful at destroying harmful molecules and preventing damage caused by some free radicals in the liver, brain and heart.
    - Basil provides protection against unwanted bacterial growth by restraining its growth.

- It improves blood flow and lessens the risk of irregular heart rhythms or a spasm of the heart muscle or a blood vessel.

NUTS

15. Walnuts: Walnut is a deeply wrinkled edible nut that is enclosed in a hard shell and a thick leathery husk and part of the tree nut family, genus Juglans. They contain omega 3-fats, copper, molybdenum, biotin, manganese among others.
    - Walnuts help fight cancer, particularly prostate cancer and breast cancer.
    - It reduces LDL "bad" cholesterol, decreases total cholesterol and increases omega-3 fatty acids in red blood cells.
    - They control aging by fighting free radicals, which are at the heart of age-related deterioration.
    - Walnuts are beneficial to male fertility.
    - They reduce the risk of excessive blood clotting by decreasing maximum platelet aggregation rate and decreasing platelet activation.

16. Almonds: Almonds are eatable brown-skinned nuts of a species of a tree native to the Middle East. They are very tasty and nutritious and used widely in cooking. Almonds have numerous benefits; they had often being used to treat a lot of illnesses. It is rich in calcium, iron, phosphorus, magnesium, vitamin B12, vitamin E, biotin and many more.
    - Almonds contain two vital brain nutrients, riboflavin and L-carnitine, which are useful in the development and health of the brain. They have also been known to reduce the risk of Alzheimer's disease.
    - It also reduces the level of LDL 'bad' cholesterol thereby reducing the risk of heart diseases.
    - The phosphorous in Almonds have been associated with the strength and durability of bones and teeth.

- Almonds have been found to be very effective protection against diabetes and cardiovascular diseases.
- Almonds are sources of alkali materials which are beneficial to the immune system that helps the body fight diseases.

EGGS

17. Eggs: Eggs are raised by female animals of different species. Some are edible and some are not. Contrary to popular belief, eggs are actually very nutritious. The old idea was that eggs were to be avoided because they are high in cholesterol. But new studies show they are actually healthy. Eggs are rich in omega 3, vitamin D, vitamin E, vitamin K, vitamin B2, vitamin B6, calcium, phosphorus and zinc. Note however that they should be eaten considerably because they still contain cholesterol, however they should not be taken out of the meal. Eggs are beneficial;
    - Eggs contain lutein, choline and antioxidants that have major benefits for eye health.
    - Eggs help increase levels of HDL, High Density Lipoprotein cholesterol (the "good" cholesterol).
    - The choline in eggs is used to build cell membranes.
    - The amino acids contained in eggs are good for general body building.

LEGUMES

18. Lentils: Lentils, a type of popular legumes, are eatable seeds that are rich in protein. The original nutrient of lentils and other legumes is protein but it has other nutrients like molybdenum, folate, fiber, copper, manganese, iron, magnesium, and some vitamins such as vitamin B1, vitamin B6, and vitamin C.
    - Lentils provide the body with energy and makes it possible to have energy while controlling blood sugar.

- Lentils help to reduce blood cholesterol since it contains high levels of soluble fiber.
- The iron in lentils is an integral component of hemoglobin, which transports oxygen from the lungs to all body cells, and is also part of key enzyme systems for energy production and metabolism.
- Lentils contain magnesium, which improves blood flow, oxygen and nutrients throughout the body.

19. Soybeans: Soybean is the oil and protein rich seed of the soybean plant native to East Asia. They are of the legume family and therefore rich in protein. They also contain iron, potassium, fiber, magnesium, sodium, Monounsaturated and Polyunsaturated fats, calcium, vitamin B6, vitamin C and many more.
   - The fiber in soybean is good for colon health and reduces the risk of colon cancer.
   - Soybeans may help alleviate the symptoms of menopause.
   - It has some bone health benefits.
   - It may also help alleviate a condition characterized by reduced bone density and increased risk of fractures, especially in elderly women.

SEA FOODS

20. Salmon: Salmon is a type of oily, edible fish in the family Salmonidae with soft fins that spends most of its life in the ocean but sometimes migrates to saltwater. Salmon has high amount of nutrients including; protein, omega 3-fats, vitamin B6, vitamin B12, vitamin D, and selenium, niacin, phosphorus, and others.
   - Salmon contain a high percentage of omega 3-fats and this nutrient have quite a lot of usefulness such as improved control of the body's inflammatory processes, better overall cell function, improved transfer of information between the body's cells, and better brain function.

- It reduces the risk and incidence of depression, hostility in young adults and cognitive decline in the elderly.
- Salmon has been found to reduce the risk of eye-related problems, especially, macular degeneration and chronic dry eye.
- It has been discovered to improve bone density and strength.

21. Sardine: Sardines are also another oily ocean fish within the herring family of Clupeidae. Sardines are also rich in omega 3-fats and protein, and they contain vitamin A, vitamin B2, vitamin B3, vitamin B12, vitamin D, sodium, potassium, selenium, choline and many more.

- The high percentage of Vitamin B12 in sardines helps promote cardiovascular well-being since it is intricately tied to keeping levels of homocysteine in balance.
- Sardines reduce inflammation, resulting in improved health, the ability to maintain proper brain function, and helping to ward off gum disease.
- They contain vitamin D which plays an essential role in bone health since it helps to increase the absorption of calcium.
- Sardines, through selenium helps prevent oxidative damage in the body, helps iodine to regulate metabolism, facilitates the process of recycling vitamin C in the body, and improves cellular function and protection.
- It also helps lighten the mood and ward off depression. Sea foods are generally very good for the body and should be seriously considered in our diet because the presence of omega 3-fats and other vital minerals and vitamins that our body needs to function well.

GRAINS

22. Brown Rice: Brown rice is whole grain rice in which the yellowish brown outer layer containing the bran remains intact. It is the best for those hoping to shed weight because it helps to reduce cholesterol in the

body. Brown rice is a good source of proteins, vitamin B3, manganese, selenium, thiamine, calcium, magnesium, fiber, and potassium.

- Brown rice provides protection against damage from the free radicals produced during energy production.
- It reduces the risk for developing chronic illnesses such as cancer, heart disease and arthritis.
- Brown rice has been found to be beneficial for postmenopausal women with high cholesterol, high blood pressure or other signs of cardiovascular disease (CVD).
- It also helps the body synthesize fats. Manganese also benefits our nervous and reproductive systems.

23. Oats: Oats, sometimes called the common oat, are the edible seeds of a species of cereal grain plant grown for its seed. Oats are consumed by humans in a variety of ways but it is also used for livestock feeding. It is loaded with vitamin B1, vitamin B6, iron, magnesium, dietary fiber, potassium, manganese, molybdenum, biotin and several others.

- Oat is a good alternative for diabetic patient and those with heart diseases because it drastically reduces cholesterol from the digestive system that would otherwise end up in the bloodstream.
- Due to the soluble fiber contained in oats, it may help reduce the risk of coronary heart disease.
- The beta-glycan oats boosts the body immune system's response to bacterial infection by completely destroying the bacteria found in an infectious area.
- Oats also helps in stabilizing blood sugar.

24. Millet: Millet is a pale, shiny grain of highly variable small-seeded grasses, widely grown around the world as cereal crops or grains for fodder and human food. It is gluten-free and full of vitamins and minerals. Millet is a rich source of vitamin B2, iron, magnesium, dietary fiber, protein, sodium, manganese, copper and numerous others.

- Millet is very rich with fiber and has low sugars. Therefore, it has a relatively low glycemic index and has been shown to produce lower blood sugar levels than wheat or rice.
- Millet reduces the severity of asthma and to reduce the frequency of migraine attacks.
- It keeps the colon properly hydrated and prevents constipation.
- Millet helps in the development and repair of body tissues.

25. Quinoa: Quinoa is the edible seed of a plant of the goosefoot family. It is not a member of the true grass family; therefore, it is a pseudo cereal, similar to buckwheat, rather than a true cereal. Quinoa is a tasty grain that is high in overall nutrients. They also contain manganese, copper, magnesium, fiber, folate, zinc and others.

- Quinoa aids the reduction of blood sugar levels, lowering cholesterol and helps with weight loss.
- It is important for health blood sugar regulation.
- Quinoa can improve metabolic health, such as lower blood sugar and triglyceride levels.
- It decreases the risk of allergies and especially perfect for people who are gluten intolerant.

HEALTHY SEEDS

1. Chia Seeds: Chia is a species of flowering plant in the mint family, Lamiaceae. It has been termed one of the healthiest foods in the world by many nutritionists and rightfully so. They are a rich source of protein, fiber, calcium, phosphorus, zinc and a host of other nutrients.

- Chia seeds are very good in reducing food craving and prevent dehydration.
- Recent studies by University of Litoral in Argentina have even linked chia seeds to the treatment of diabetes, by curing the causes of diabetes.

- They are a great source of strength. It was originally used by the ancient Aztec warriors, to boost energy. And in fact, chia means, "strength" in Mayan language.
- The antioxidants in chia seeds fight the production of free radicals, which can damage molecules in cells and contribute to ageing and diseases like cancer.
- They are also good for the skin.

2. Flaxseeds: Flax is a food and fiber crop. Flaxseeds are the small brown or golden colored seeds of the flax and they are sometimes called, linseed.
   - They help reduce sugar craving and thereby promote weight loss.
   - The antioxidant benefits of flaxseeds have long been associated with prevention of cardiovascular diseases and have recently also been tied to decreased insulin resistance.
   - It helps beautify and freshens the hair and skin by reducing dryness and flakiness.
   - Mucilage, contained in flaxseeds supports the intestines during digestion by improving absorption of certain nutrients in the small intestine.
   - Flaxseeds also help decrease cholesterol in the body through its soluble fiber content.

3. Sunflower seeds: Sunflower seeds are the edible seeds gotten from tall annual sunflower plant. Sunflower seeds are very good alternative of a snack instead of unhealthy junks. They are very rich in vitamin E, calcium, selenium, vitamin B1, magnesium, phosphorous, a lot of other vitamins and healthy monounsaturated and polyunsaturated fats.
   - The healthy monounsaturated and polyunsaturated fats lowers the risk of cardiovascular diseases.
   - They also serve as building blocks for cell membranes and allow the body to balance hormones.

- It has been discovered that the magnesium contained in sunflower seeds help reduce the severity of asthma, lower high blood pressure, and prevent migraine headaches.
- Sunflower seed is a good source of vitamin E and Vitamin E helps guard the cells against tough chemicals that oxidize and damage proteins, cell membranes and DNA in the body.
- Selenium in the sunflower seed improves detoxification and helps prevent cancer.

4. Pumpkin seeds: Pumpkin seed is simply the edible seed of a pumpkin. It contains protein, potassium, sodium, magnesium, vitamin A, iron, zinc and many more.
    - Pumpkin seeds help to ensure good sleep.
    - They help regulate blood pressure and help prevent sudden cardiac arrest, heart attack, and stroke.
    - Pumpkin seeds are known for their anti-microbial benefits, including their anti-fungal and anti-viral properties.
    - They improve insulin regulation in diabetic patients and also prevent some unwanted consequences of diabetes on kidney function.
    - They have been discovered to be beneficial for men and used for the treatment of mild Prostatic Hyperplasia (BPH).

5. Sesame seeds: Sesame is the small oval white seed of the sesame plant of the family of the genus Sesamum. Sesame seed is a source of copper, manganese, magnesium, zinc, folic acid, iron, molybdenum, selenium and so on.
    - Sesame seed may help prevent coronary artery disease, and stroke by favoring healthy serum lipid profile.
    - It lowers cholesterol level, prevents high blood pressure and increase vitamin E supplies in the body.
    - Sesame seed contains folic acid, a nutrient good for pregnant women as it may prevent neural tube defects in the newborns.
    - It has also been discovered to protect the liver from oxidative damage.

- It provides structure, strength and elasticity in blood vessels, bones and joints and serves as relief for Rheumatoid Arthritis.

6. Mustard seeds: Mustard seed is the small, round, and pungent seed of a brassica plant. It is rich in vitamin B6, vitamin C, magnesium, iron, dietary fiber, calcium, polyunsaturated fat and monounsaturated fat, omega 3-fats, selenium, manganese among others.
   - B-complex vitamins found in mustard seed help in enzyme synthesis, nervous system function and regulating body metabolism.
   - Mustard seed has been found to hinder the development of existing cancer cells and to be protective against the formation of such cells.
   - It maintains the integrity of cell membrane of mucus membranes and skin by protecting it from harmful oxygen-free radicals.
   - Mustard seed helps to reduce the severity of asthma, to lessen high blood pressure, to decrease the regularity of migraine attacks, and to avert heart attack in patients suffering from atherosclerosis or diabetic heart disease.

7. Coriander seeds: Coriander seeds, also called cilantro, are the edible seeds of an aromatic plant of the family Apiaceae. It contains vitamin A, vitamin B6, vitamin C, magnesium, potassium, protein, and more nutrients.
   - Coriander seeds are relatively valuable in alleviating countless skin diseases like itchy skin, rashes, eczema, and inflammation.
   - They help stimulate the secretion of insulin and lower blood sugar.
   - Coriander seeds contain dietary fiber as well as antioxidant properties that promote the healthy operation of the liver and aid bowel movements.
   - It contains an antibacterial compound that could demonstrate to be a safe, natural means of combating Salmonella, a recurrent and occasionally terminal cause of foodborne illness.
   - It reduces the amount of LDL "bad" cholesterol and increases the amount of HDL "good" cholesterol in the blood.

8. Cumin seeds: Cumin seeds are the aromatic seeds of a plant of the carrot family Apiaceae. Cumin seeds are also listed among the world healthiest food because of the wealth of nutrients it contains. The seed is a rich source of vitamin A, vitamin B6, vitamin C, iron, magnesium, calcium, sodium, potassium,

    •   Cumin seeds act as an antioxidant to fight the free radicals that affect the skin and trigger symptoms of ageing like wrinkles, age spots and flabby skin.

    •   The full iron in cumin seeds helps transport oxygen from the lungs to all body cells, and is also part of key enzyme systems for energy production and metabolism.

    •   They are also a good source of dietary fiber which helps in the cleaning process and removes toxin.

    •   Cumin may fuel the exudation of pancreatic enzymes, compounds essential for appropriate digestion and nutrient absorption.

    •   They also help to lower blood sugar levels and thus help in maintaining proper blood content levels in the body.

FOOD SUPPLEMENTS

Food supplement, from the term is the additional nutrients included in our diet in case of deficiency. They are the nutrients or even diet that may otherwise not be consumed in sufficient quantities. They usually come in form of pills, tablets, capsules or liquids in measured doses, so they are not food in the real sense of it. They are more like nutrients administered to correct nutritional deficiencies or sustain satisfactory consumption of some nutrients. Some of the most popular include but not limited to: multivitamins and minerals, omega 3-fats, calcium, creatine, enzyme complex, Glucosamine and Chondroitin,

1. Multivitamins and Minerals: Daily intake of multivitamins and minerals has been popular termed the insurance against the plethora of nutritional deficiencies caused by washed-out important nutrients in the soil, through pollution, food processing, pharmaceuticals, and chronic diseases. The standard dosage is usually one per day and taken

with meal, but it is better to see the doctor so as to be sure of the proper dosage depending on individual peculiarities. It is a good supplement and in fact, should be considered compulsory for pregnant women as it may protect the fetus from any heart defects. It has also being known to increase intelligence. Additional, it is useful for boosting the immune system.

2. Fish oil and Omega 3-fats: Omega 3 is prominent in fish and although it is found in plant food sources, it is prevalent in animals like fish. Fish oil also consists of other kind of oil called the EPA (eicosapentaenoic acid) and DHA (docosahexaenoic acid). And it is another supplement that might be necessary depending on factors that erode nutrients before it gets to the final consumer. The nutrients in fish oil are used in the treatment of many health issues such as, diabetes, ADHD, Alzheimer's disease, inflammatory bowel disease, anxiety, depression, high cholesterol, heart disease, arthritis, eczema, cancer, weakened immunity, autoimmune disease and macular degeneration. Again, it is useful for the proper improvement and performance of the brain, where it helps brain cells transmit electrical impulses efficiently.

3. Calcium: although calcium can be found in popular foods that we eat like fish, raisin, beans etc., it has been discovered that this nutrient is one of the nutrients that people have deficiency on. About 1000 to 1200mg of calcium is recommended for an adult and calcium lactate or nitrate are usually the best alternative to go for but again, it is usually better if it is diagnosed by the doctor. The heart, muscles and nerves also need calcium to function properly. Calcium is very important for the prevention of osteoporosis because its deficiency is one of the major factors that cause osteoporosis. And popularly, calcium is useful for the development and maintenance of strong bones.

4. Creatine: Creatine is a nitrogenous biological acid formed in the liver that aids the provision of energy to cells all over the body. Creatine is created of three amino acids: L-arginine, glycine and L-methionine and forms about one volume of the complete volume of the blood in our body. The supplement is available in both powder and tablet form. One of the benefits of creatine is that it enhances brain function and

also quickens recovery. Additionally, it is good for sport as it increases muscle strength.

5. Enzyme Complex: Enzyme as commonly known is like a catalyst that produces a metabolic reaction in the body. The body therefore needs the adequate amount of enzymes that would keep the body functioning properly. The enzymes are of various forms and they all have their individual benefits. The important thing though is that enzymes propel the organic processes required for the body to develop natural resources in the system, distribute nutrients, eradicate undesirable chemicals, and a plethora of other biochemical processes that take place in the body. Enzymes have been known to be valuable for some cases of cancer, especially pancreatic cancer. In addition, enzymes have been found useful in the treatment of chronic digestive problems such as colitis or irritable bowel syndrome because it enhances food digestion and absorption.

6. Glucosamine and Chondroitin: Glucosamine is a natural substance gotten from animal tissues such as crab or shrimp shells and Chondroitin sulfate is contained in animal cartilage such as tracheas or shark cartilage. They both have individual functions but most times, they come as complex, a combination of both drugs. They provide significant relief from osteoarthritis knee pain. Chondroitin is a main element of the connective tissue in the body known as cartilage, which helps pad the joints and prevent friction of the bones.

7. Ashwagandha: Ashwagandha better known as the Indian ginseng has been used for centuries as a cure and as a healthy diet. It is a very nourishing herb and the herb has a wide range of activity that promotes physical and mental health, body rejuvenation, and longevity. Though it is forbidden to pregnant women, it has been found as a good supplement. The recommended dosage is usually 250 mg to 500mg daily. However, doctors' orders are still the best. Ashwagandha's antioxidant ability helps to enhance memory and improve brain function. It has also been shown to stimulate red blood cell production, especially in children to improve anemia. Furthermore, it has been lauded as an anti-depressant considering it helps reduce stress.

8. Green Tea: Green tea is usually one of the first things that come to mind when people want to lose weight but it actually has more benefits than that. It has been discovered that those who take green tea on a regular basis appear to have less incidence of cancer. Green tea consumption was associated with a decreased risk of lymph node metastasis in premenopausal women with cancer, reduced risk of breast, lung, stomach, prostate, colon, esophagus, skin, bladder, liver, oral leukoplakia, ovary and leukemia, cancer. Green tea also improves brain function, and as mentioned earlier perfect for weight loss.

9. Vitamin C: Vitamin C, also known as Ascorbic acid is a water soluble vitamin found in most fruits and vegetables. It has various benefits ranging from its value to the skin and the popular help in reducing the complications that could be gotten from common cold. Many fruits contain vitamin C and should be incorporated in our meal. But most of these nutrients are lost even in fruits because of the fertilizers used to grow them or because of environment, pollution and all other limitations. However, some would still be retained or better still, if we can find where we can buy fresh fruits. Be as it may, vitamin C is a crucial factor necessary for the production of collagen, a protein found in the connective tissues of the body. It provides protection against immune system deficiency. It is further important for the prevention and treatment of scurvy; and the prevention of wrinkling and other signs of aging.

10. Vitamin D: Also called "THE SUNSHINE VITAMIN" though popular is actually in low quantity in most of our diets and it is necessary to replenish in order to avoid some diseases. Sufficient vitamin D consumption is vital for the control of phosphorus and calcium, maintenance of bones and teeth, and has been found to provide protection against numerous diseases and conditions such as cancer and type 1 diabetes. Vitamin D can also lift our moods, cheer us up and help those that are in the weight loss journey melt stubborn pounds.

ONE SIZE FITS ALL

Nutrient standard DOES NOT really seem to be the best way to establish the nutrient needs for a diverse population. A common folly is to assume a 'single multiple' Vitamin product will provide you with all key nutrients but this is not the case. Unless the multivitamin were the size of a golf ball it would be unable to provide optimal doses of each Vitamin and Mineral.

Realistically, we need OPTIMAL DOSES OF 4 DIETARY SUPPLEMENTS, for instance, a multivitamin, a Vitamin C product, a Vitamin E product, and a multi-mineral product.

IMPORTANCE OF AMINO ACIDS

HEY, I NEED MY AMINOS! That is your body speaking, complaining about running low on amino acids.

Our body contains proteins, about 20 percent of it in fact. Protein plays a vital role in our body and amino acids are the building block of the protein. A large portion of our body – cells, muscles and tissues – contains amino acids. It is very important in providing structure to our cells and ultimately our body

There are 14 nonessential amino acids that the body can manufacture & of course our body needs them & manufactures them as long as it receives sufficient quantity of the 8 essential amino acids. So this is how it goes - The body can't manufacture the 8 essential amino acids as they can't be stored as fats, therefore must be supplied to the body through food and supplements. Not having enough of the 8 can affect the body's metabolism; they are used in biosynthesis of protein. A simple way to remember the 8 essential amino acids when you need to is through the acronym "TV UNTIL PM" (as in watching TV until Late at night. The 8 super amino acids are; Tryptophan, Valine, Threonine, Isoleucine, Leucine, Lysine, Phenylalanine, and Methionine.

Tryptophan is needed for the prevention of illnesses and even death. Food sources include fish, sesame seeds, spirulina, bananas, peanuts, oats, buckwheat, almonds, sunflower seeds, pumpkin seeds and salmon.

Valine is necessary for enhancing our immune system, improving our nervous system and healing of insomnia.

FOOD SOURCES: fish, beans, mushrooms, whole grains, cheese, soy beans, nuts and seeds, and many more.

Threonine improves the immune system by helping the body create antibodies to fight diseases. It also helps strengthen the bones and produce muscle tissues.

FOOD SOURCES: liver, lean beef, cheese, beans, and dairy foods. Isoleucine is used to promote normal growth of the body and help regulate blood sugar. Sources include soy, rye, cheese, almonds, cashew, lamb, egg, fish and many more.

Leucine prompts muscle growth and it is known specially for playing regulatory roles in the metabolism.

FOOD SOURCES: seafood, soy beans, chicken, beans, seeds and nuts. Lysine helps the body absorb calcium from the intestinal tracts and it also promotes bone growth.

FOOD SOURCES: peas, cheese, sardines, eggs, lean meat, soy beans and others.

Phenylalanine has been associated with the treatment of depression and it is essential for the central nervous system to function properly.

FOOD SOURCES: soybean flour, milk, eggs, cheese, spinach, amaranth leaves, lean beef, lupin seeds among others.

Methionine is used to break down fats in the body and it is also a major source of sulfur.

FOOD SOURCES: meat, fish, sesame seeds, Brazil nuts and so on.

BCAA: BCAA is an acronym for Branched Chain Amino Acids. It is a term used to describe the amino acids that have similar structures. The amino acids are Leucine, Isoleucine and Valine. Their functions as a whole cannot be overemphasized as can be seen above. Together, they can be found in seafood and lean meat (lean because red meat can be dangerous when taken in excess. So it is necessary we remember to take them moderately and also opt for the safer version). It is important to note that the deficiency of these supplementary foods can be harmful to the body.

However, the overdose can also be counterproductive.

So it would be wise not to get too enthusiastic in the usage. The wisest decision is getting a doctor's prescription because that would be given with individual peculiarities in consideration.

Do you want to look great and feel great? Never miss out on your greens! Do you want a flawless complexion? Get rid of acidity? Feel active and vibrant? Stay young? If your answer is YES, the solution is simple

NEVER MISS OUT ON YOUR SALADS – GO GREEN FEEL GREEN!

All the foods listed above are counted among the healthiest foods in the world and should not be taken with levity; however, there is still a lot to be said about vegetables. Salads are loaded with vitamins and minerals such as: vitamin A (immunity), vitamin C (fight infection, boost iron absorption, maintain healthy bones, gums and skin), vitamin K (strong bones, heal wounds, assists blood to clot), calcium (build strong teeth and bones, assists blood to clot, nerves to carry messages, muscles to contract), alpha- and beta- carotene (antioxidant that help protect against cancer and heart disease), iron (maintain healthy blood) and many other vitamins and minerals.

Nourishment of the skin and to get that healthy glow is the need of the hour. To keep your skin healthy and your face looking great, make sure you have a generous portion of salad leaves & GREEN FOODS every day. My daily salad intake includes Iceberg lettuce & WHOLE LOT OF OTHER GREENS Spinach, kale, rocket leaves with light dressing, AND please avoid the thousand island and high calorie dressings as you are sure to defeat the purpose of eating greens. When you fill up your salad with dressing, you might as well not eat greens because the purpose of healthy living would be defeated in that instance.

On the final analysis, sleep is a very important lifestyle to imbibe in keeping our body nourished and far from diseases. Sleep is no longer a waste of time as formerly believed. It is also a necessary part of our body process.

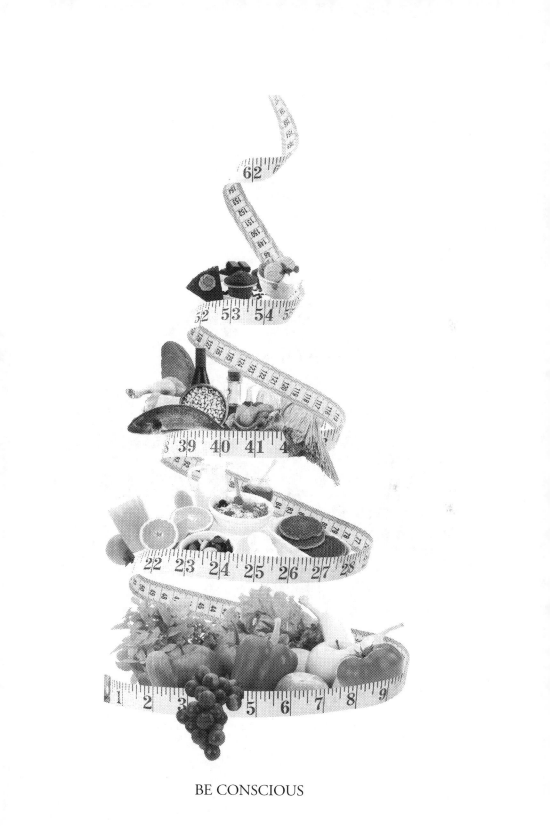

BE CONSCIOUS

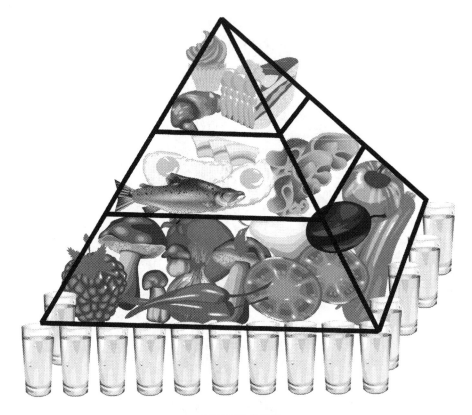

BELLY OFF!

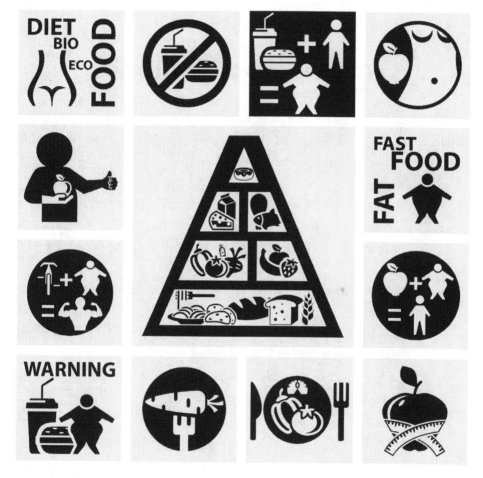

YOUR SCALE WILL TELL THE TALE!

Chapter Seven

A Few Food Demons

Having explained super foods and their benefits, there is a need to explain the effects of bad foods on our body.

1. White Sugar: White sugar is popularly known as refined sugar and it is generally harmful. Some of its effects include;
    *   It contains no essential nutrients and therefore useless to the body.
    *   White sugar feeds cancer cells in the body.
    *   Sugar increases one's blood sugar, thereby increasing the risk of diabetes.
    *   It is one of the major reasons for weight gain and obesity and we all know what they ultimately result to.
    *   White sugar can BE HIGHLY DAMAGING & can overload the liver, and can cause liver diseases.
    *   SIMPLE SOULTION: Just don't go "OVERBOARD" with that Sugar-Urge!!!!

2. White Rice: White rice doesn't contain as much nutrients as brown rice and it is also generally unhealthy. So it is advisable to substitute brown rice for white rice because;
    *   White rice increases the risk of diabetes.
    *   It increases the risk of obesity.
    *   It causes accumulation of fats in the body.

3. MILK: Yes, Milk CAN HAVE ITS SIDE EFFECTS

4. This is due to the fact that milk:
    - can increase the risk of Cancer
    - elevates estrogen levels
    - has also been found to increase the risk of diabetes.
    - One side effect of white milk is eczema and acne.
    - It has been discovered to promote premature aging, allergies, IBS (irritable bowel syndrome) and more

5. White bread: As delicious as white bread is, it is additionally a meal that we are advised to avoid or at least take in small quantity.
    - White bread seriously increases the blood sugar level because of how fast it is digested and absorbed in the body.
    - White bread has being refined and therefore has lost most of the nutrients that should have otherwise been there.
    - It increases weight and causes obesity.
    - It increases the risk of diabetes and heart diseases.
    - It has been discovered to cause mood swings and bouts of depression.

We can see from the above that it is indeed better to embrace brown grains and whole grain foods in place of white foods in general. White foods are indeed very delicious and they call to us often, but the real purpose of food is to nourish us and if it is not nourishing us, then we should do away with it.

Chapter Eight

A Simple Formula for Healthy Living: 70% Kitchen, 30% Exercise

We have been talking about diet and how much it affects our health and rightly so. All the meals mentioned above are just a fraction of the meals we can take and we would not have to worry our pretty little heads about diseases. There is a lot of meals we can take without feeling guilty that we are punishing our body. These meals are aromatic, tasty and best of all nutritious. However, as we are eating right, we need to also exercise right.

Exercises are like the backbone of healthy living. One of the fastest ways of losing weight is when diet is combined with exercises and as a matter of fact, it is the surest way. Other methods which are shortcuts would get you there first but reprisal is almost sure in such cases. If you want something long-lasting, which is also healthy, then you really have to step up your game and change your lifestyle. Indeed, the best chance at living healthy is seventy percent kitchen, thirty percent lifestyle and exercises. This simply means while it is important to look into your kitchen and do away with foods that are dangerous to your health and introducing healthy ones, it is equally important to look into changing one's lifestyle and incorporating a lot of exercises in order to get maximum results. *Remember Abs is made in the Kitchen & Sculpted in the Gym*! The importance of both factors to our health cannot be overemphasized.

Exercises are simply physical activities intended to improve health, strength or fitness. Exercises are also defined by Encarta dictionary as physical activities and MOVEMENTS, especially when intended to keep a person fit and healthy. From the above definitions, we can see that some things are clear, which are, exercises are physical, exercises can be movements, and they are intended for health and fitness. It is needless to say exercise is very important. And luckily we do not necessarily have to register in a gym and make everything formal. We could always make it fun by engaging in physical activities with friends and family, do more house chores instead of relying on a machine or just find every opportunity to move the body around, instead of living sedentarily.

It is AMAZING AND SHOCKING the number of times I see people taking the lift even if it is to go up one floor, they would rather wait a few minutes (Sometimes up to 10 minutes –Yes I've timed this as an exercise to gauge human self-love or lack of it & luckily for me they don't even know I'm there) for the lift than simply walk up a floor or two. This is the kind of guy who is slacking big time.

We then complain about health issues, tubby stomachs, diabetes and so on. Motivate and shift the mind into making yourself the lean machine "YOU ARE MEANT TO BE"

Cardio is really vital and should be engaged in by every human. Just running up the stairs alone strengthens your heart and lungs, reduces high blood pressure, improves blood cholesterol, and you may say Good Bye to developing Type 2 diabetes. The running stairs workout really strengthens the same muscles as lunges and squats, and works on your lungs and heart. You are basically forced to work against gravity. And that is just running up the stairs; imagine the benefits you would accrue from getting serious about all other activities.

There is a lot of exercises that you could partake of, some of which you would need a gym to accomplish and others you can do at home. They range from Triceps (back of arms) and Biceps (front of arms), Squat, Leg press, Standing calf raise, Seated calf raise, Deadlift, Leg extension, Leg curl, Wall Sit, Hamstrings (back of legs), Snatch, Pectorals (chest), Lats (mid back), Deltoids (shoulders), Good-morning, Push up, Shoulder Press, Pull down, Russian Twist, Dive-bombers, Bear Crawls, Lunges and many more.

Also, there are different classifications or types of exercises that a lot of people do not know about. Most people just concentrate on a type of exercise and think they are good to go. But for maximum results and prevention of injuries, it is usually necessary to mix it up. The four main types of exercises are; endurance, strength, flexibility, and balance.

ENDURANCE EXERCISES: Endurance exercises which are also called aerobics refer to exercises that involve or improve oxygen consumption by the body. Aerobics actually means 'having or providing oxygen,' and refer to the use of oxygen in the body's metabolic or energy-generating process. They keep your heart, lungs, and circulatory system healthy and improve your overall fitness. Doing aerobics make it easier to carry out many of our everyday activities and have a different intensity than other types of exercises. They include, cycling, brisk walking, hiking, swimming, rowing, skipping rope, and other low intensity exercises.

BENEFITS OF ENDURANCE EXERCISES

- Endurance exercises improve the body's immune system by producing additional proteins essential for the creation of white blood cells and antibodies.
- Endurance training also encourages faster metabolisms due to more lean muscle mass.
- It improves the body's sensitivity to insulin, thereby helping with the prevention of diabetes.
- Endurance exercise improves blood circulation throughout the body, thereby also boosting the activities of all vital organs in the body, such as the brain and heart.

STRENGTH EXERCISES: Strength exercises are usually anaerobic (having or providing no oxygen) can firm, strengthen, and tone muscles, as well as improve bone strength, balance, and coordination. They boost power and develop muscle mass. Muscles trained under anaerobic exercises build up differently, bringing about improved performance in short duration, high intensity activities. They are a lot more intensified than the endurance exercises and they exert more energy. Even small upsurge in strength can make a distinct difference in our ability to stay independent and carry out everyday activities, such as climbing stair cases and carrying heavy items. This type of exercise include; pushups, weight lifting, bicep curls, sprinting, lunges etc.

BENEFITS OF STRENGTH EXERCISES

- Strength exercises are the best form of exercises for losing weight. It is very effective because it not only loses the weight but maintains the weight loss.
- Also, as the term implies, it increases the muscle strength and gives the body enough strength for the rainy day.
- It protects and prevents loss of bone and muscle mass.
- It aids the body in the prevention and control of chronic conditions such as heart disease, arthritis, diabetes, back pain, obesity and depression.

BE A RUBBERBAND MAN –Just Stretch, it's Imperative & a Simply Fantastic Feeling Challenge Yourself/Anti-Age – BE CONSCIOUS!

STRETCHING & FLEXIBILITY EXERCISES: Flexibility is quite explicit and it is a vital but often disregarded classification of exercises. As the term implies, it include exercises aimed at lengthening and stretching muscles. Exercises such as stretching help to enhance joint flexibility and keep muscles limber. The objective is to develop the range of motion which can decrease the possibility of injury. Being flexible gives you more freedom of movement for other exercises as well as for your everyday activities. Some examples of flexibility include but not limited to yoga, upper body stretch, back stretch, back of leg stretch and many more.

BENEFITS OF FLEXIBILITY EXERCISES

- Flexibility has been known to improve all kinds of posture and especially helps the body after exercises; it improves muscular balance and resting posture.
- Flexibility exercises help prevent injuries, back pain, and balance issues.
- It boosts the supply of blood to muscle tissues, and the entire body distributing necessary nutrients across the blood stream.

- Flexibility exercises can also be a good way to start the day as it helps the body relax.

BALANCE EXERCISES: Balance is the most uncommon of all types of exercises. But they are useful for helping us stay balanced. They are used to help us maintain our balance at any age and are mostly used for older people to keep them from losing balance and preventing too much dependence on the younger generation to move around. Virtually all activities that keep you on your feet and moving, such as walking, can help you maintain good balance. But precise workouts intended to improve your balance are valuable to embrace in your regular practice and it can help enhance your stability. They consist of Tai Chi, leg swing, one-legged balance, heel-to-toe walk among others.

BENEFITS OF BALANCE EXERCISES

- Balance exercises are good for us because as we get older when we no longer have that much stamina, the exercises accumulated over the years keeps us from embarrassing falls.
- It keeps the body agile.
- Balance exercises are good exercises to employ for toning the thigh and hip muscles.
- It also helps in stabilizing the joints and developing coordination of the body generally.

From the above, we can see that all the categories of exercises are beneficial and we should not ignore any of them. A proper exercise would be one that involves one or two of all categorizations.

BENEFITS OF EXERCISES

Exercises have its value to the health and it goes beyond weight loss contrary to popular belief. It also goes a long way in saving us from doctor's visit. Some of the benefits of exercises include;

- Frequent exercises have been associated to the reduction of diseases like cancer and diabetes by about 50 percent and early death by about 30 percent.
- Exercises improve the sleep quality of insomnia patients.
- Regular exercises can improve your thinking, learning, and judgment skills and also reduce the risk of having depression.
- Exercises keep your self-confidence on an all-time high. Not only would you feel good about how you look physically, it is would also psychologically lift up your mood.
- It reinforces the muscles that are involved in respiratory exercises and enables the movement of air in and out of the lungs.
- It boosts high-density lipoprotein (HDL) "good" cholesterol and decreases low-density lipoprotein (LDL) "bad" cholesterol and unhealthy triglycerides.
- Frequent exercises can boost your muscle strength and improve your endurance level.
- It also helps with the skin in that it gives it an improved complexion and keeps it toned.
- It keeps the body out of stress by reversing the effect of stress.
- And finally, regular exercises are essential to imbibe because it reduces drastically, if combined with healthy diet, the risk of almost all chronic diseases, such as diabetes, cancer, dementia, heart diseases, cardio vascular diseases and many others.

BENEFITS OF YOGA

Yoga is very flexible breathing exercises and postures that can be traced to Hindu yoga. Some of its benefits include;

- It brings about improved concentration.
- It is a flexible exercise and therefore makes you flexible.
- Yoga teaches you better ways of dealing with stress.
- It makes it easier for our blood to flow round our body.
- Yoga improves general health and keeps one in perfect health.

MAKE MR DUMBELL YOUR FRIEND - BENEFITS OF WEIGHT TRAINING

- It gives the body optimal strength. If you have being battling with weakness and carrying those bags of groceries, now might be the time to invest on some weight training.
- Weight training can improve your health because it works with your lungs and heart.
- You also lose those extra flabs and weight that you have been struggling with, with weight training.
- Weight training helps build bone mass and reduce bone problems.
- It also gives you confidence.

BENEFITS OF PILATES

- Pilates elongates, strengthens and improve the bones.
- It also helps make us more stable as it gives us balance.
- It is very good for weight loss and body toning.
- It boosts our stamina and gives us better posture.
- It has been discovered as a good treatment for back pain.

DONT IGNORE YOUR LEGS - RESPECT THEM!

I have always wondered why many men ignore training their legs – a big reason is that they do not wear shorts and feel if the upper body looks good that is enough of an endorsement to say, "I am fit and I am buff enough." But the real deal is to have great powerful legs and I do not necessarily mean ripped body builder legs, but a powerful foundation that could be achieved through sports, running or kick boxing. Legs are biggest muscle group in the body and we should maximize them.

BENEFITS

- It helps the release of growth hormones.
- Exercising the legs accelerates fat loss.

- It is good for upper body improvement.
- Leg exercises enhance body symmetry - as a big upper body and toothpick legs look ridiculous.
- It improves mental strength.
- It increases testosterone levels

PSYCHOLOGICAL BENEFITS OF INVOLVING CHILDREN IN SPORTS

A lot of parents probably want to see their children involved in sports in school because of how proud it makes them (the parents) feel. And some parents have an aberration to sport because they want their children to have their head buried in books always. But the truth is sport is very beneficial for the general development of the child and that is what the parents should be concentrating on. Parents should groom their children into sport activities in their formative years because;

- Getting involved in sporting activities gives children a sense of belonging. It makes them feel accepted by their peers.
- It boosts their self-esteem because sports increase their well-being generally. So when they feel good about themselves, it helps their esteem.
- It teaches them teamwork and decreases the feelings of selfishness or self-centeredness. Sports involve working together with others to achieve a common goal and that would prepare them for the future.
- It reduces stress and depression. One of the greatest causes of depression in children and adolescents is lack of a sense of belonging. But when they are accepted and feel like they are doing something that matters, it improves their mood and prevents depression.
- It would improve their mental concentration and keep their brains sharp.

TRAIN ME BUT KNOW ME FIRST –KNOW YOUR TRAINER

This might sound unnecessary because you might be thinking "what do I need to know my trainer for? After all, all I need is the work." But you couldn't be more wrong. You have to know your fitness trainer. Your fitness trainer is like your teacher just that in this case, it is for your body. The same way you need to know your teacher to have a maximum relationship with him/her is the same way you should make it a point of duty to know your trainer. Don't be apprehensive to ask questions, you have a right to have questions or even concerns and have them settled. Also, don't just agree with whatever he says, cross-question him if you have to, just make sure you feel comfortable about going on with the training. Don't get forced into training excessively, remember you know your body, listen to your body signals. Many trainers force grueling schedules on their clients without actually understanding their lifestyle, nutrition, sleep patterns, and stress levels. Some of them forget they are experts and it didn't take them a day to get there. So they might want to make experts out of their clients just too soon. Be vocal and make any discomfort you have known.

It is equally important that you get the right trainer who is certified by a recognized fitness body and who is part of a well chain of health clubs etc. that are stringent on screening their employees and fitness nutritionists trainers.

A fitness trainer should inspire you. I personally don't get inspired by trainers who are not in great shape and who don't know. You cannot give what you do not have. A teacher that is empty has no business being in a classroom; therefore it might be difficult to find inspiration from a fitness trainer that is not fit.

Chapter Nine

Are Your Hormones Causing You Havoc?

"WHEN ADAM BECOMES MADAM & EVE BECOMES STEVE"

There are many instances where people who should otherwise be alright have raging hormones affecting them. Almost like the case of people with allergies, what should be good to eat and what is considered healthy for others might affect them because of their hormones. Hormones and hormonal changes differ, especially as relates to gender. We have Testosterone (male hormone), Estrogen (female Hormone), Progesterone, Serotonin, Dopamine and others.

TESTOSTERONE is secreted primarily by men. It helps in maintaining muscle mass, bone density, and sex characteristics. For the male to function properly as a male, his testosterone has to be adequate and secreted properly. A deficiency and too much of it could pose a problem. However, the level of this hormone naturally reduces as a man advances in age, mostly from age 30. Raging hormones can cause low self-esteem, eating disorder, depression and many other vices in people. This could be as a result of growing too fast or not growing enough with peers. And it can be corrected through diet. Eating meals that contain zinc such as beans, cheese, seafood, pumpkin seeds, coconut, wheat bran, strawberries and vitamin D such as sunlight can really help. Exercises have also been found to be helpful with hormonal issues.

ESTROGEN is found mostly in females and is a primary female hormone. It is associated with the development and regulation of the female reproductive system and secondary sex characteristics. It is produced by the ovaries and naturally reduces when a woman starts undergoing menopause. Blood sugar level, breast cancer can be because of high level of hormones present in the body. And when they are absent or lesser than the body needs, it could also bring about havoc to the health. Although different hormone therapies have been tried to help women but it is usually better to check the diet first. A healthy diet which consists of food like dates, apricot, flax seed, sesame seeds, beans, chickpeas, peas, alfalfa sprouts and soy, and regular exercises would do you a world of good in calming raging hormones.

PROGESTERONE is also a female hormone secreted by the ovaries mostly for controlling menstruation and maintaining pregnancy. When it is too much, it can cause PMS (premenstrual syndrome). It can also cause problems when it is not enough in the body. This is because progesterone and estrogen complement each other in the body. Progesterone counters the effects of estrogen and estrogen does the same thing to progesterone. To control progesterone, food with high sugar should be reduced and foods like seafood, bananas, spinach, beans, potatoes, berries, watermelon, crabs, spinach, okra and pumpkin should be eaten. Don't forget your regular exercise; they help balance your hormones.

DOPAMINE is a transmitter in our brain that controls reward. It makes us see the reward of particular actions and move towards achieving those rewards. People who are risk takers have a higher level of it. When we experience lack of motivation, focus, hopelessness, and sometimes addiction to different vices as a way of trying to get motivation from something else, it is an indication that we do not have enough dopamine in our system. And the best way to rectify this is through balanced diet and regular exercises. Fruits such, leafy greens, oats, yoghurt are good to boost our dopamine level.

SEROTONIN is also a neurotransmitter in our brains that smooth our muscles and regulates our body processes that are associated with making us happy and well. So naturally, when we do not have enough of it in the body, it can cause depression. For increase, some people use therapies, but the best method is still eating food with high level of serotonin and exercising adequately. Foods such as walnuts, hickory nuts, pineapple, bananas, kiwis, plums, tomatoes and serotonin boosting foods like turmeric, green tea, chocolate, and fish. The most effective method has been found to be combining healthy carbs like rice, oatmeal and tryptophan rich foods like salmon, lentil, poultry food, cheese, nuts and seeds.

OXYTOXIN is one of our hormones that help with child birth and male reproductive organ. In females, it is the hormone that helps women with everything that has to do with child delivery including contractions during labor and in males; it has a huge role to play in the ability of a man to reproduce. Just like the other hormones, if it is too low or too high, it causes problem. And just like above, the best remedy is diet; avoiding foods like high saturated foods that increase your stress level, eating meals like happy fruits that improve your mood and regular exercising to make you feel good about yourself. Interestingly, experts have also discovered that being affectionate, feeling loved and doing a good deed balances the oxytocin level in our body.

We can see from the above that our diet and our hormones are interrelated just like our diet affects every other thing that goes on in our body. It would do us a world of good, especially when we are aging and all these hormones are raging and causing havoc to revisit our diet, they usually work better than artificially taking in these hormones. We should not also forget our exercises and the need to stay stress-free as much as we can, so we can keep living without hormonal issues.

Chapter Ten

Definition of Concepts

CHOLESTEROL AND TRIGLYCERIDES

Cholesterol is quite popular and it has being recurring right from the start of this book because of how involved it is with our health as regards nutrition. It is actually gotten from the combination of two Greek words, chole (bile) and stereos (solid). It is known by the scientists as a steroid alcohol sterol made by the liver and present in all animal cells because it is an essential structural component of all animal cell membranes that is required to maintain both membrane structural integrity and fluidity. Despite the entire gist we have heard about how we should flee from cholesterol, cholesterol is really vital to the body as an integral part of our cell membranes, and is involved in the formation of bile acid and some hormones.

FUNCTIONS OF CHOLESTEROL

Some of the functions of cholesterol include;

- It aids the building and maintenance of membranes
- Cholesterol plays a part in producing hormones such as estrogen, testosterone, progesterone, aldosterone and cortisone.
- It has been discovered that cholesterol may serve as an antioxidant in the body.
- It is important for the production and synthesis of vitamin D.

- Cholesterol produces bile acids which aid in digestion and vitamin absorption.

I hope we can clearly see that cholesterol is not all bad as we have been made to believe, after all even the body produces cholesterol of its own. However the problem starts when it is too much in the body. Excess cholesterol in the blood can increase one's chances of getting circulatory or heart diseases. So it needs to be checked in order not to be too much. But it is also not supposed to be deficient.

GOOD AND BAD CHOLESTEROL

You have probably being reading about the good and bad cholesterol and wondering what they mean. Cholesterol moves around your bloodstream in small bundles known as lipoproteins. These bundles are made of fat (lipid) on the inside and proteins on the outside. There are two kinds of lipoproteins that carry cholesterol throughout your body; they include the Low Density Lipoproteins (LDL) and High Density Lipoproteins (HDL). Although the LDL is often known as the bad cholesterol, having healthy levels of both types of lipoproteins is important.

High Density Lipoprotein HDL is called the good cholesterol because it is protective. It carries cholesterol from other parts of your body back to your liver and the liver removes the cholesterol from your body, thereby ridding the body of excess.

Low Density Lipoprotein on the other hand is termed bad because of its unhealthy process. A high LDL level leads to a buildup of cholesterol in your arteries, thereby blocking the movement of blood that normally goes on in the arteries. The arteries are blood vessels that transport blood from the heart to the whole body.

DIAGNOSIS AND TREATMENT

So how do you know when you have a high LDL level? It is simple. You go for the test and get tested for it because usually it doesn't show any signs till it escalate into more serious diseases. Drugs could be administered for treatment but usually, the best preventive and even curative method is introducing diet with high HDL cholesterol and low the LDL cholesterol; and regular exercises.

TRIGLYCERIDES

Triglyceride is another word we hear and cower. You need not worry, you would learn all about it in just a few minutes. This big scientific word is gotten from a combination of three fatty acids (tri) and glycerol (glyceride). It is an ester formed from a molecule of glycerol and three molecules of fatty acids. We have being told it has serious effects on human health when consumed in excessive amounts.

FUNCTIONS OF TRIGLYCERIDE

The main function of triglyceride is the provision of energy to the body. As a matter of fact, without triglyceride in the body, you would lose energy except if you are eating constantly, an alternative that is also not good for your weight. When you take in more calories than your body need, it gathers and stores those calories in the form of triglycerides. Fat cells hold the triglyceride molecules until your body needs energy, especially between meals. Your hormones inform the fat cells to release the triglycerides when your body needs energy.

However, excess triglyceride also has issues in the body. It causes heart diseases and cancer. Doctors advise a triglyceride level of 150 milligrams per deciliter or less to reduce one's chances of heart disease. Some of the factors that cause triglyceride are usually diet high in carbohydrates and low in protein, Cirrhosis or liver damage, disorder passed down through family.

Just like high cholesterol can be treated with drugs, high triglycerides can also be treated with drugs. However, the best method is still exercises and healthy diet: reduced calories and more fruits and vegetables.

BLOOD PRESSURE

Blood pressure is the pressure applied on the walls of blood vessels when the blood is circulating round the body. Blood pressure can either be high or low depending on the pressure of the blood against the wall of the arteries as the heart pumps blood. When one's blood pressure is low, it is called hypotension and when it is high, it is called hypertension.

You determine your blood pressure by going to the medical practitioners to get tested. They test you using a gauge, stethoscope or electronic sensor, and a blood pressure cuff. Blood pressure readings have two numbers, written as a ratio. A number is usually on top and the other lower number. The number on top is called the systolic blood pressure while the lower number is called the diastolic blood pressure. The systolic blood pressure is when the heart beats while pumping blood and the diastolic blood pressure is when the heart is at rest between beats. The reading for a normal blood pressure is 90 to 120 systolic and 60 to 80 diastolic. Anything less is hypotension and higher than that is hypertension.

HYPOTENSION

Most of us have probably not heard of hypotension because it is very rare compared to hypertension. Hypotension as mentioned earlier is a situation where by the force of the blood on the wall of the blood vessels during blood pump is lower than normal. It is determined by blood pressure that is found to be less than 90/60. It is not much of a disease but a physiological state because on its own, it might not need to be treated in most healthy people but sometimes, it could be indicating an underlying problem.

Hypotension could be brought about by a number of factors, such as low blood volume, hormonal changes, widening of blood vessels, medicine side effects, anemia, heart problems or endocrine problems. Low blood volume or hypovolemia is the most common situation that could be as a result of dehydration, starvation, hemorrhage, diarrhea or vomiting.

Hypotension (Low Blood pressure) usually doesn't give people signs but in a severe case, the person may experience lightheadedness, fainting, unconsciousness, seizure, irregular heartbeat, among others and drugs can be used to correct the situation.

HYPERTENSION

Hypertension (High Blood Pressure) is the most risky one and the one we all hear of. It is a root cause for a lot of chronic diseases and it can cause death. It is usually caused by a sedentary lifestyle; a salt-rich diet associated with processed and fatty food, and alcohol and tobacco use. All these usually do not depict themselves till when one is growing old, and then the effects start rearing its ugly head. That is why you hardly find cases of hypertension in young people.

- Hypertension is a situation where the blood pressure reads higher than 90/60. But normally, it is in stages;
- 120 to 139 systolic and 80 to 89 diastolic – prehypertension stage.
- 140 to 159 systolic and 90 to 99 diastolic – hypertension stage one.
- 169 or higher systolic and 100 or higher diastolic – hypertension stage two.
- Higher than 160 systolic and higher than 110 diastolic – emergency case.

High blood pressure is very dangerous as it can result to a lot of issues on its own. It is closely related to stroke, cardiac arrest, coronary disease, kidney failure, to mention but a few. Experts have let us know that blood pressure increase with age and size due to accumulated plagues in the blood stream. But I am sure we already understand considering what we have been emphasizing that proper diets would help reduce the risk of both high and low blood pressure and the proper exercise will keep the blood flowing smoothly.

RHEUMATOID ARTHRITIS

I am sure we have heard of different cases of arthritis, especially as relates to older people. Some of us are probably wondering what it is all about and we have the answer here for you. Rheumatoid arthritis is an autoimmune condition, which means it is caused by the body's immune system attacking itself. You know the immune system is like the soldiers that help us fight germs in the body. Now imagine if those soldiers start destroying what they are supposed to be protecting, that is what rheumatoid arthritis is all about. Although it usually happens with the joints, it does not just affect the joint in some people; the disease could also damage a wide variety of body systems, including the skin, eyes, lungs, heart and blood vessels.

CAUSES OF RHEUMATOID ARTHRITIS

It is still much of a mystery to our doctors what exactly prompts the immune system attacking itself. However, they have also discovered a number of things that could contribute to the risk of getting the disease; genes, smoking, hormones (especially in the cases with women because of the production of estrogen), obesity, bacterial infection and exposure to air pollution of any kind. A larger percentage of people suffering from rheumatoid arthritis are women; that is why it is linked with estrogen production.

SYMPTOMS AND TREATMENT OF RHEUMATOID ARTHRITIS

A cure for the disease has not been found but it can be managed to prevent complications when discovered; although it could take weeks to discover its presence. The symptoms usually range from tender or swollen joints, soreness and pain, redness, stiffness, weight loss in some cases. The severe cases in other parts of the body could be dryness in the affected area, irritation, small lumps and pain. If one discovers all the symptoms, rush to the doctor and the doctor would most likely administer Disease-modifying anti-rheumatic drugs (DMARDs), anti-inflammatory drugs, steroids, or surgery for people with permanent damage. Also if you find yourself with rheumatoid arthritis, you might want to invest in anti-inflammatory diet such as cold-water fish like tuna, salmon, herring; fruits; vegetables; whole grains; olive oil and avoid as much as possible salty foods, smoking or indirect smoking, alcohol, and sugar. Also, aerobics and strength training would be very beneficial in strengthening the bones and reducing pains in patients.

ASTHMA

Asthma is a very popular disease as it has no restriction on age or gender. Even some babies are diagnosed with asthma. Asthma concentrates on the lungs and the airways in the body.

Asthma is a chronic disease involving the airways in the lungs. These airways, or bronchial tubes (in scientific terms), allow air to come in and out of the lungs. It is a respiratory condition that is caused by shrinking of the bronchi of the lungs, resulting in difficulty in breathing. It is usually connected to allergic reaction or other forms of hypersensitivity that causes infection of the airways. The airways of the patient swells and whenever there is a trigger, the muscles around the airways tighten, restricting the movement of air in and out of the lungs.

CAUSES OF ASTHMA

Most people try to conceive what exactly causes asthma. Asthma has been said to be caused by contact with airborne allergens (substances that causes allergies) during childhood, inherited from parents with asthma, viral infection during childhood, respiratory infection during childhood. Don't be surprised most of the causes relate to happenings during infancy and childhood. This is why most cases of asthma are discovered at infancy or early ages.

But asthma unlike most sickness can be passive except if it comes in contact with factors that triggers it. What happens is the carrier would have it and it would not necessarily hamper that person's life, however when the person comes in contact with factors like cold, strenuous exercise, dust, smoke, it could further tighten the airways and make it more difficult to breathe. Asthma can be contained and in some cases, can cause death if it is not attended to.

SYMPTOMS AND TREATMENT OF ASTHMA

There is still no cure for asthma. What is important is that you make sure you find a doctor once you notice the symptoms which is sneezing, wheezing, coughing, chest tightness, shortness of breath, etc. The best known treatment is avoiding the triggers as much as possible, taking medication and using inhaler when you start feeling signs of an attack.

Also remember to go for regular checkups so as to determine how regular the asthma attack is. This process is done through what is called a Peak Flow Meter (a small, hand-held device that would show you how well air moves out of your lungs. You blow into the device and it provides you with your peak flow number that lets you know how your lungs are working at the time of the test).

ATHEROSCLEROSIS

Atherosclerosis is a disease of the arteries caused by the buildup of plaques of fatty materials on its walls, resulting to hardening and narrowing of the arteries. And what happens as a result is that the movement of blood and oxygen to the organs of the body do not move as they are supposed to. I hope you know arteries are like pipes where blood and all other good nutrients flow round the body. Normally, arteries are flexible and elastic, after some time, because of the gathering of undigested fats and macrophage white blood cells in the walls of the arteries, the walls of the arteries can become hard in a condition commonly called hardening. Atherosclerosis can be dangerous because sometimes the plaques can burst causing a blood clot (thick blood) in the body and it could also lead to heart attacks or stroke and even death.

CAUSES OF ATHEROSCLEROSIS

The main cause of atherosclerosis is when the LDL 'bad' cholesterol gathers in the arteries and the body sends macrophage white blood cells to remove the bad cholesterol from the body but instead of doing just that, the white blood cells might get stuck in duty. Then, walls of the arteries would now have a combination of the fats and the macrophage white blood cells. Now imagine when the pipe connected to your kitchen tap where water passes freely usually now gets filled with some materials that restrict the flow of the water. The water will not flow as freely as before and lesser volume will come out of your kitchen tap. That is exactly what happens here, the restriction of blood affects the flow of blood to vital organs that need it for the proper running of the body.

Other external factors that causes atherosclerosis include; high sugar content in the body, smoking, high LDL 'bad' cholesterol content in the body, high level of triglycerides, high blood pressure, inflammation caused by the presence of other diseases, unhealthy diet and lack of exercise.

SYMPTOMS OF ATHEROSCLEROSIS

The symptoms that a person feels when he or she has atherosclerosis are usually weakness, leg pain, numbness, headache, chest pain, shortness of breath, loss of appetite, sleep problems and others. If you feel these symptoms, it is important to visit a doctor immediately. Atherosclerosis usually occurs at old age but accumulation starts from childhood.

Atherosclerosis has been found to be possibly prevented by;

- Eating heart healthy food which would consist of less of saturated fats and more of fruits and vegetables (including beans and peas), whole grains, lean meats, poultry without skin, seafood, and fat-free or low-fat milk and dairy products.
- Engaging in physical activities and exercises.
- Quit smoking, directly or indirectly.

TREATMENT OF ATHEROSCLEROSIS

However, if one already has the disease, it could be treated through the following mediums;

- Lifestyle Change: This is probably the best way and should still be imbibed as a complement to the other treatment. Changing from unhealthy diet to heart healthy diet is very important to battling atherosclerosis. Make sure to include fruits, legumes, vegetables, whole grains, fat free dietary products, fish oil instead of saturated oil and stay away from red meat, foods with saturated fats, palm and coconut oil, smoking, and sugary foods. Then be more involved in physical activities, engage in intentional exercises instead of living sedentarily.

- Medication: The doctor may prescribe statin medicine like to control or lower cholesterol, anti-platelets to help prevent blood clots or medications to prevent the buildup of plaque. Remember however that as you take your medicines judiciously; don't neglect keeping a healthy lifestyle.
- Surgery: Surgery could also be prescribed for more advanced cases. Medical surgery procedures such as coronary angioplasty, coronary artery bypass grafting (CABG), and carotid endarterectomy can go a long way to help treat atherosclerosis.

ANGINA

Angina is a problem of the chest. The chest experiences pain, pressure, squeezing, tightness or just general discomfort caused by reduced flow of oxygen-rich blood to the heart muscle. The pain can also spread to your shoulders, arms, neck, jaw, or back. Plus, sometimes, angina may even feel like indigestion. Angina is not a disease on its own but a symptom of more serious diseases such as coronary heart disease. That is why it is important to visit the doctor once you notice this feeling, so as to detect any other issue and tackle it early. Angina attacks usually occur when one uses so much energy and therefore needs more oxygen than the blood supplies to the heart.

CAUSES OF ANGINA

Angina is caused mainly when the arteries narrow or harden because of the accumulation of fats and macrophage white blood cells in the walls of the arteries. The macrophage white blood cells were sent to wade off the LDL cholesterol but it instead, gets stuck. This therefore affects the blood that the heart muscle receives; the reaction to this deficiency is what causes angina. Remember the explanation of the water pipe and your kitchen tap? That is exactly what happens here as well. Some external factors are what contributes to the materials that block the arteries and they are; unhealthy diet, unhealthy cholesterol level, unhealthy triglyceride level, sedentary lifestyle, smoking, high blood pressure, old age, stress, and family history of heart disease.

SYMPTOMS OF ANGINA

The symptoms that one is likely to feel with angina is chest pain or just general discomfort, pain in the shoulders, arms, jaw or back, dizziness, fatigue, cramping, heart burn, and shortness of breath. As usual, if you feel any of these issues, make sure you quickly visit the hospital.

TREATMENT OF ANGINA

The doctor after testing to be sure it is an angina and not a usual chest pain would most likely prescribe;

- Lifestyle changes of reducing foods with saturated fats, sugary foods and junks and substituting them with heart healthy diets like fruits, vegetables, legumes, avoiding smoking, living a stress-free life while also incorporating physical activities.
- In some really severe cases, surgery procedures like angioplasty can be used to also correct the reduced flow of blood to the heart muscles.

LUPUS

Lupus is a chronic, autoimmune, inflammatory disease that occurs when your body immune system attacks your own tissues and organs. What happens with lupus is that the immune system which is supposed to help the body fight diseases instead fights the body it is supposed to be protecting and cause damage in the body. I am sure you can still recall the example of soldiers destroying where they are supposed to be protecting, same thing happens here. Normally, the immune system produces proteins called antibodies that protect the body from diseases. So what happens in this case is that the body immune system is unable to recognize the difference between harmful organisms and some body tissues, and then secret some unusual antibodies to tackle the body tissues causing inflammation, pain and damage in the affected area of the body. Lupus cannot be cured but treatments can be administered to help control symptoms. Additionally, lupus cannot be contacted nor is it related to having cancer in anyway. Lupus is also more common in women of childbearing age and usually occurs between the ages of 15 to 40.

CAUSES OF LUPUS

Some people are prone to developing lupus because of some hereditary factors, and others may be brought about by infections, certain medications and ultraviolet light.

SYMPTOMS OF LUPUS

It has been continually said that lupus is really hard to identify because most of the symptoms resemble that of many other illnesses. However lupus has a signature sign of a butterfly looking rash on the face that covers the cheeks and bridge of the nose and it is accompanied by fatigue, hair loss, loss of appetite, headache, fever, photosensitivity, eye dryness, chest pain and shortness of breath.

TREATMENT OF LUPUS

Sun screens, sun protection clothing, sun avoidance should also be imbibed. Healthy diets and exercises as well as adequate rest are advised for people suffering from lupus.

DIABETES

Diabetes, known by doctors as 'Diabetes Mellitus' is a group of metabolic diseases in which there are high blood sugar levels as a result of absence or inadequate production of insulin, or inability of the body to properly use the insulin over a prolonged period. Normally, insulin is a hormone produced in the pancreas that controls the level of glucose in the blood. Patients with high blood sugar will become increasingly thirsty (polydipsia), experience frequent urination (polyuria) and hunger (polyphagia). In 2013, according to the Williams' textbook of endocrinology, it was estimated that over 382 million people throughout the world had diabetes.

Diabetes is divided into three types;

- Type 1 Diabetes: It was formerly known as 'juvenile diabetes' because it was common among children, and young adults or insulin-dependent diabetes. In this case, the body does not produce insulin at all. Luckily, only about 10% of the people with diabetes suffer from this diabetes type 1.
- Type 2 Diabetes: This is usually called 'non-insulin-dependent diabetes.' Most cases of diabetes are type 2 diabetes. For this type of diabetes, the body does not produce enough insulin to properly breakdown the sugar and control the glucose level in the body.
- Gestational Diabetes: This usually happens to women during pregnancy. In this case, women who have very high levels of glucose in their blood, and their bodies are unable to produce enough insulin to move all of the glucose into their cells, and this gradually increase the level of glucose in their body.

CAUSES OF DIABETES

The cause of diabetes, all the types, is mainly as a result of insulin and its inability to adequately regulate glucose in the blood. But the risk factors of diabetes include family history, sugary foods, environmental factors such as exposure to certain viral illnesses, overweight, and sedentary lifestyle.

SYMPTOMS OF DIABETES

Symptoms include; frequent urine, frequent thirst, weight loss, hunger, fatigue, yeast infections, blurred vision, hunger, and numbness. Once these symptoms are seen, the best thing would be to visit the doctor.

TREATMENT OF DIABETES

Diabetes mellitus cannot be cured but they can be managed. And while type 1 cannot be prevented, type 2 diabetes can be prevented to some extent with healthy lifestyle and exercises. Type 1 diabetes is managed by administering insulin, engaging in exercise, and a diabetic diet. The first step to treating type 2 diabetes on the other hand is usually weight reduction; then a type 2 diabetic diet, and exercise. Additionally, sugar and carbs should be greatly reduced.

CONCLUSION

In conclusion, we all know it is not enough to have information, it is usually more important to act on it. That is why wisdom is of more value than knowledge, knowledge is just information and in our advanced world today, getting knowledge is usually just at the click of a button but applying that knowledge is what differentiates us from others. So having learnt all these information, please IMPLEMENT IT, AND DON'T JUST SIT ON IT! That is the only way we can all together create a disease- free and healthy world. Diet, exercises and health are totally interrelated. If you followed judiciously, you would discover that there is hardly any of the illnesses or diseases that did not require a form of lifestyle change or the other. And the dominant lifestyle changes were usually diet and exercises. I am sure we do not need a seer to tell us what we need to know and it is not rocket science to figure out at this point that the only way to stay away from diseases is to eat the right things at the right time and involve yourself in adequate exercises.

BE CONSCIOUS (Recommended) DIET

The BE CONSCIOUS Diet has been devised to energize the human body and maintain optimum PH Levels

Foods known as "White Poison" should be eliminated from the BE CONSCIOUS Diet. These are, refined flour (Maida), White Rice, Sugar, Milk. Avoid all kinds of Saturated and Trans fats as they are highly acidic, fattening and slow down the metabolic rate, causing Arthritis amongst other diseases that lead to ill health.

Essentials:

Early Morning:
- ❖ Herbal tea *
- ❖ A glass of green juice **
- ❖ Soaked nuts (5 almonds with 1 date or 1 fig and 3 walnuts)
- ❖ 1 bowl of fruit with Black Salt – Watermelon is a must, Papaya, Chickoo (Sapodilla or Sapota) or Banana
- ❖ 1 tsp soaked seeds (Sunflower, Pumpkin, Flax and Sesame with a bit of Gojiberries)

On days when you are still hungry, you may have a small bowl of:
- ❖ Millet flakes cooked the same way as Poha (flattened or beaten rice) or Upma (Semolina)
- ❖ Cereal (Spelt flakes, Puffed Amaranth etc.) with coconut milk or Almond Milk

Mid-Morning Options:

- ❖ Light Buttermilk made with Jeera (cumin), ginger and mint leaves. You can have up to 5 glasses, before 5 30 PM.
- ❖ Lime juice with mint Leaves and Black Salt.

Lunch: (Cold pressed oils must be used to cook. The oil must be added to the Dal, or vegetables after the vegetables/Dal(lentils) are in the cooking Pot/ Pan not before as the oil must not be smoked or heated directly)

- ❖ Please refer to the list of BE CONSCIOUS recommended foods. They can be combined and cooked in a way desired by you.
- ❖ As Quinoa, Millets, Brown rice and Buckwheat and Dalia (Broken wheat) are filling, it will not leave you hungry for more, so the quantity is not restricted.
- ❖ Wheat Pasta or Noodles can also be cooked for lunch.

Dinner: Soup – Clear or thick (without corn flour) Salad (boiled/Steamed Vegetables, grilled chicken or grilled fish)

BE CONSCIOUS OF:

Foods to be avoided: Breads & Yeast products.

In Moderation: Daal (Black gram lentils) & Channa(Chickpeas), (soaked for at least half an hour before cooking), Peanuts, Sooji, Kaali Daal,(Black gram lentils) Rajma (Kidney beans) Jaggery, Coffee, Tea, Eggs, chicken, fish, fruits.

Unlimited quantities: Leafy greens, Asparagus, lime, lemons, Avocados, Sprouts, Coconut and Watermelon (unless diabetic)

Herbal tea: 2 Cups of water with Ginger, Pudina (Mint 5 leaves) Tulsi (Basil 5 leaves) boiled and reduced to 1 glass, Can add a bit of Jaggery to this.

Make a Super food Green Juice: 1-2 teaspoon of Wheat grass powder, Parsley, Cucumber, Lettuce, Spinach, Celery. Beat well with a little water and drink immediately with lime juice to taste.

BE CONSCIOUS FEEL ALIVE!

Printed in the United States
By Bookmasters